# LIFE
# WITHOUT
# PAIN

# LIFE WITHOUT PAIN

*Free Yourself from Chronic Back Pain,*
*Headache, Arthritis Pain, and More,*
*without Surgery or Narcotic Drugs*

RICHARD M. LINCHITZ, M.D.

**ADDISON-WESLEY PUBLISHING COMPANY, INC.**

Reading, Massachusetts   Menlo Park, California   New York
Don Mills, Ontario   Wokingham, England   Amsterdam   Bonn   Sydney
Singapore   Tokyo   Madrid   Bogotá   Santiago   San Juan

**Library of Congress Cataloging-in-Publication Data**

Linchitz, Richard M.
  Life without pain.

  Bibliography: p.
  Includes index.
  1. Intractable pain—Treatment.  I. Title.
RB127.L455   1988       616'.0472       87-19360
ISBN 0-201-11900-5

Jacket photograph and design by Martucci Studio
Text design by Anna Post
Set in 10-point Cheltenham by Compset, Inc., Beverly, MA
Line drawings by Charles Egri and David Minard

ABCDEFGHIJ-D0-8987
First printing, December 1987

*To my wife, Rita, and my children,*
*Elise, Michael, and Jonathan*

# Contents

# PART III: PUTTING YOUR CHRONIC-PAIN-CONTROL PROGRAM TO WORK

# LIFE
# WITHOUT
# PAIN

# PART ONE

# UNDERSTANDING
# THE PROBLEM

# 1

# The Worst Pain

If you're a victim of chronic pain only you know how it feels. No one else can ever fully comprehend your individual discomfort and frustration no matter how hard they try—not your doctor, not your family, nor any of the people who love you and want to help you. The lesson we learn from life is that pain is experienced alone. It cuts you off from others, and it makes your body feel like a prison.

This book is dedicated to breaking down that prison wall, and the first thing you the reader should know is that you're not really alone at all. Ironically, as many as 65 million Americans may be suffering the isolation of chronic pain, each in his or her own way. Over half the American population has backaches, and more than 10 percent experience serious back pain at least thirty days a year. Three fourths of Americans have headaches; a good 15 percent of them are chronic headache sufferers. Pain, *the* major cause of visits to physicians, represents a cost to the nation's economy of between $70 and $90 billion a year in medical expenses and lost productivity.

Despite the scope of the problem, those of us who study chronic pain and work with its victims every day have some surprisingly good news to offer —good news in the form of powerful new techniques to bring pain under control. Unfortunately, it takes time to spread the word. Of all statistics on pain, the most unsettling to me is that 18 percent of the people reporting pain they considered severe or unbearable had not even consulted a health care professional because they felt that nothing could be done.

Fifteen years ago such pessimism might have been justified, because the alternatives then available to patients were not very inspiring. There was surgery, which offered risk and the prospect of further pain, and there were drugs, which could lead to depression and dependency. A third alternative consisted of the humiliation of being told, "It's all in your head." If it didn't show up on the test, it wasn't there.

But now we can all give thanks that the situation has changed dramatically. New, integrated approaches to pain therapy developed in just the last few years have helped literally thousands of people overcome their pain and resume living their lives without narcotic drugs and invasive surgical techniques. Drawing on my own clinical experience, I have gathered a constellation of techniques, ranging from deep relaxation to guided imagery to exercise, to put into this book for you to use at home.

In my clinic, the Pain Alleviation Center in Roslyn, New York, we see people from all walks of life, ranging in occupation from housewives to professional baseball players. These patients often come to us because they've been frustrated elsewhere. Because their pain hasn't yielded to any one therapeutic approach, they're ready for something different—a totally comprehensive pain-control program.

At the center, our patients benefit from the combined wisdom and training of a complete team of health care professionals—specialists in physical medicine and rehabilitation, nutrition, physical therapy, psychology, and even dentistry—working together to arrive at an effective, individualized therapeutic regimen. This same approach, the same team effort, lies at the heart of *Life Without Pain*.

As director of the center, as a psychiatrist, and as a physician specializing in the total care of chronic-pain patients, I play my most important role in leading the team to meet individually with each patient, to counsel, to guide, and to give all of them the background understanding they will need to become active participants in their own recovery. I have made the same effort in the organization of this book.

My first objective has been to provide a very simple but useful grasp of the basic anatomy and physiology of pain. In my experience, this background helps the patient tremendously in understanding the therapies we advise. I want you to understand some of the reasoning behind our advice, because we truly want you to become a full partner in turning your life around.

The problems we treat at the center are not just an occasional ache or pain. Our patients are people in serious distress. One woman, for instance, had such severe headaches that she could no longer speak coherently. She wove in and out when she walked and tripped over her own feet. She'd had these migraines every day for ten years—3,650 days in a row.

Another woman who came to see us was seriously considering suicide because of the pain of rheumatoid arthritis. The pain had begun mildly enough in a knee and a finger, but then it spread to other joints. By the time she arrived at the Pain Alleviation Center, it simply never let up.

Then there was the man who had been bench-pressing three hundred pounds; then seven muscles popped loose from his upper back, seven ligaments tore away from his spine, and other ligaments that cemented his spine to his ribs and upper back gave way. Even though he had undergone three operations, he said the pain was still like having hatchets in his upper back for twenty-four hours a day, and it had been like that for thirteen years.

Recent research has shown, and our clinical experience demonstrates, that chronic pain is a unique and multifaceted syndrome, a disorder that affects whole lives rather than just joints and muscles. This awareness of the personal context of pain, which is central to our approach, is something I learned many years ago while I was in training at the University of California at San Francisco Medical Center. My wife was working as a nurse, assisting a team of neurosurgeons who treated severe chronic pain by putting implants in the brain and severing nerves. Wondering what could possibly drive people to submit to such extreme measures, I began interviewing some of these patients. I gained a certain insight into what they were suffering, but I also learned the intense frustration of simply being a chronic-pain patient—being shunted from one specialist to another, being told, "You'll just have to live with it," being cut off from work and family life and from the pleasure of the most ordinary activities. That was when I became convinced of the need for an approach that would be as fully integrated into the patients' daily existence as were the problems that I saw.

I began an extensive search of the literature of pain. Already trained as a psychiatrist, I began to read the reports of neuroscientists and others who were unraveling the answers to the most basic questions of what pain is and how it is conveyed through the body. I became immersed in the research findings of the National Institute of Neurological and Communicative Disorders and Stroke (NINCDS), the National Institute of Mental Health (NIMH), the National Institute of Dental Research (NIDR), and the National Cancer Institute (NCI). I also became affiliated with the International Association for the Study of Pain and the American Pain Society and studied the significant contributions they have made to the theory and practice of chronic-pain control.

I found a series of giant strides toward a safe and effective therapy for alleviating chronic pain, the key elements of which include:

- a new upgraded evaluation of the usefulness of some of Eastern medicine's pain-control practices—deep relaxation and acupuncture, for example
- a new emphasis on physical exercise, from calisthenics to jogging and swimming, to manage stress and pain
- a new understanding of the roles certain nutrients, mainly amino acids and vitamins, play in fighting pain and depression
- a new wave of milestone discoveries by neurobiologists—scientists who study the brain—that have pinpointed the brain's natural painkillers, the endorphins.
- a new grasp of chronic pain as a disease shaped in part by factors traditional medicine had not previously considered—the family, the workplace, the social environment

After finishing my residency, I returned to Long Island and established my practice, focusing on the care of chronic-pain patients. Very quickly, though, I became frustrated with the limitations of a single practitioner trying to treat patients with such varied problems and needs. Many of the people I saw were seriously depressed by their pain, but they were also depressed by the disruption of their lives. To make matters worse, they were suffering significant overall physical weakness as a result of their inactivity, having lost muscle tone and cardiovascular conditioning. All too frequently they were addicted to narcotic analgesics and/or sedative hypnotic drugs, and just as frequently they had seen their family relationships deteriorate, leaving anger and resentment between themselves and their loved ones.

In time, the solo practice of Richard Linchitz, M.D., evolved into the Pain Alleviation Center, a multispecialty clinic whose staff included, besides me, another physician specializing in physical medicine and rehabilitation, behavioral psychologists, a dentist specializing in temporomandibular joint syndrome and facial pain, physical therapists, a movement therapist, and an acupuncturist. We now provide a new comprehensive concept of pain care: the "total pain-control program," a therapy that integrates all the major advances and the best that traditional medicine offers into a single regimen that is as effective as it is doable.

# THE TOTAL PAIN-CONTROL PROGRAM

At the Pain Alleviation Center, therapy begins with my evaluation of the patient and his or her complaint. This encounter links the traditional physical examination with new techniques (the thermogram for example, which helps diagnose the actual cause of chronic pain of "unknown origin") and with an assessment of the emotional, social, and psychological influences on the disease.

We then work out a regimen for each patient that may include some of the more successful traditional therapies with the best of the new therapies, including those which will become part of your pain-control program:

- *Drug management.* A simple technique, using what we call the "pain capsule" to break the narcotic-analgesic/sedative drug habit
- *Biofeedback,* with which you measure stress reduction in your body while you feel the accompanying relief of pain
- *Total relaxation techniques,* based on breath control and mind control, which fight stress and pain
- *Self-hypnosis,* with which you can direct your pain to stop
- *Autogenics,* a technique that triggers the brain's pain-relief mechanism
- *Guided imagery*—movies of the mind—which activates the brain's pain-relief mechanism with mental images
- *Movement therapy*—exercises anybody can do—for muscular relaxation leading to the production of endorphins, the brain's painkillers
- *Nutrient supplements,* to fight depression and pain
- *Diet,* to boost the manufacture of endorphins and improve overall health
- *Life enhancement,* to learn how to live with others while you're conquering your pain and to help others live with you

The wonderful thing about these therapies is that you can learn how to use them without the support of a pain-control center, although you may prefer to have it. A complete program that has worked for others, your pain-control program, starts on page 33.

This program should be supervised by a physician trained and experienced in chronic-pain control. Before you begin the program, you should obtain the approval of your supervising physician, and while you follow the program you should have your supervising physician monitor your progress regularly.

## TYPES OF PAIN TREATABLE THROUGH YOUR PAIN-CONTROL PROGRAM

Remember that your pain-control program treats pain only. It does not treat the diseases, like arthritis or cancer, that cause pain. For such treatment you should consult your doctor. It is sometimes necessary to supplement your pain-control program with clinical therapy, and certainly you should follow the advice of the physician supervising your program.

The type of chronic pain from which you suffer probably appears on the following list.

Abdominal
Angina
Ankle
Arthritic (rheumatoid
    arthritis and
    osteoarthritis)
Back (upper and lower)
Bursitis
Cancer
Cancer treatment
    (from chemotherapy
    and radiation)
Chest
Dystrophy (causalgia)
Fibrositis
Fibromyalgia
Foot
Gout
Hand (including that of
    Raynaud's disease)
Headache
Hip
Kidney
Migraine
Myofascial pain syndrome
Myofibrositis
Neck (including
    spondylolisthesis)
Neuralgia
Neuroma (caused by tumors
    on nerve ends)
Phantom (such as the pain
    of a limb that has
    been amputated)
Postoperative
Sciatic
Shingles (herpes zoster)
Stomach
Systemic (pain throughout
    your system)
Tendinitis
Tennis elbow
Trigeminal neuralgia (tic
    douloureux), known as tic

The fundamental distinction you should remember is that ordinary pain, called acute pain, yields to medical treatment or to the body's own superlative healing apparatus within six months. Chronic pain is designed never to yield. It can come from ongoing damage—from cancer, from interstitial cystitis, from ear infection—in which the relatively short-term signals of acute pain that alert you to injury persist, pile up, and are transformed into the intensities of chronic pain. Or it can come from injury—a ruptured disk, perhaps—in which the pain remains as if it were a memory long after the damage has healed. In still other cases, it comes from no known cause.

For me chronic pain—and the sudden role-reversal of becoming a chronic-pain patient—came quite by surprise after years and years of my engaging in vigorous physical activity. A longtime competitive triathlete, I awoke one morning after a hundred-mile bicycle race with the shocking realization that part of my right leg had become paralyzed. It didn't take long for me to come up with a possible diagnosis—a herniated disk in my lower back, a condition that could cause paralysis by pressing one of the spinal nerves. But even with my medical training and intellectual grasp of what might be happening, I refused at first to accept the truth. I even tried to "work through" the pain, going out to run with a bland smile on my face, limping through the neighborhood as if nothing was wrong.

After two days the pain forced me to overcome my denial, and in time I saw a neurologist and neurosurgeon who advised me to watch for any worsening signs and to take "absolute bed rest" for two weeks. I tried to be a good patient, but the back pain steadily worsened as my motor strength deteriorated. It was then that this nightmare became a true learning experience for me as a physician.

As bad as the pain was, the worst aspect for me was the growing and quite depressing sense that my days of vigorous exercise were over. My doctor began ruling out, one by one, the very activities— running, bicycling, weight lifting—that had become a part of my identity since early adolescence. Despite all the consolations I was told to remember—my career, my lovely wife and family—the sense of loss was overwhelming, and I was completely devastated.

As you might imagine, however, the story doesn't end there. After weeks of depression and soul-searching, I experienced a profound and interesting transformation. I simply decided to take charge of my life once again. I accepted that "for now" I was indeed unable to participate in sports as I had always enjoyed them. I made peace with my limitation, but from that moment on I resolved never to doubt that I would come back. I gave myself no specific deadlines or time frames. But what truly astonished me was the extent to which my simple decision began to make me feel better. Not physically, at first. The pain was still there, but the sadness had begun to lift and was replaced by a calmer acceptance of the present and a hope for the future. I began to realize that I was taking the same first emotional steps I encourage my patients to take, the first internal steps toward recovery.

Over the next year I followed the very program we administer at the Pain Alleviation Center. By no means the best of patients, I became discouraged at times. Sometimes I pushed myself too hard, and sometimes I held myself back. I did not pay attention to my body signals at every opportunity, but overall I followed our program and, in fact, succeeded. I began using the progressive resistance exercise machines at the center, starting with virtually no weight when only a short time earlier I had been lifting hundreds of pounds. I began swimming again on a regular basis but for much shorter distances and with much less intensity. After a couple of months, having built back some of the strength I'd lost in my right leg, I added walking to my program of recuperation. Then I began to swim in a new way, taking the opportunity of my relative inactivity in other sports to concentrate on improving my strokes.

I also found that during this period of recuperation I was spending more time with my family and enjoying that time more than ever. In fact, I found myself saying the same things I'd heard my patients say after going through our program: that in a strange way this experience of overcoming chronic pain was an opportunity to learn things about myself, to explore my limitations and failings, and to find new strength and a new sense of achievement.

Each person's experience with pain and recovery is, of course, quite different. We all have different things to gain and to lose, to fear and to hope for. But my own encounter with chronic pain has given me a much deeper empathy toward my patients and a strong conviction that the methods outlined in this book have real value. I firmly believe that this value can extend past the goal of reducing suffering and that it can reach into the realm of improving your life, your self-esteem, and your sense of personal fulfillment.

# 2

# The New Hope

If you and I were sitting in my office for your first patient interview, I would probably begin by explaining that in spite of the long history of medicine, only recently have scientists come to understand how pain works. With this new knowledge, specialists have now devised ways of controlling how pain is turned on and off. You will learn to use these techniques in the chapters ahead.

To give you some understanding of this knowledge, however, we need to take a brief look at the most extraordinary creation in the universe, the human brain. We need to explore what it's made of, and to watch its chemistry in operation. Hardly more than a decade ago we wouldn't have had even the vocabulary to describe the process—that's how new this knowledge is.

Why must you understand how the brain works? Because in reading this book you'll learn to manipulate your brain to make it work against your pain. If you don't believe you can do it—and for pain sufferers it may sound too good to be true—you won't try it. Then you will lose the chance of enjoying the bright new hopes in pain medicine. Your belief in the exceptional uses of your brain is the key to controlling your pain.

We all learned in school that the brain and nervous system comprise the communications network for the body, but what we couldn't have known then is that there are biochemical substances which carry the body's internal communications. Each of these substances, which are called *neurotransmitters,* carries a different type of message.

Some of them transmit pain, and they are the ones known, appropriately enough, as *substance P.*

Fortunately, other newly discovered messengers act as blockers of pain, and these have been given the name *endorphins,* which means simply "the morphine within." These pain-blocking messengers are the neurotransmitters with which you'll be most concerned as you learn to control your own sensations of pain.

To understand these "on" and "off" switches for pain, let's look a little more closely at the basic units of the brain, the brain cells or *neurons.* Each one has an antenna-like structure sticking out from its nucleus. These antennae are called *dendrites,* and they receive messages from neurotransmitters into the neurons.

When your nerves are stimulated by something which is causing harm to your body—a sharp object on your finger, for instance—they send signals up the spinal cord to the brain. These signals are carried by the neurotransmitters called substance P.

At the top of the spinal cord the substance P reaches the neurons of the brain. To continue its progress, it must be received by the dendrites of some neuron, but each dendrite receptor will accept only certain types of neurotransmitters. In the appropriate receptor, substance P will fit like a key in a lock. In the others, it will not fit at all.

When substance P is received by a neuron's dendrites, it causes that neuron to "fire," sending out a fusillade of biochemicals that includes more substance P. This new substance P, in turn, can fit other neurons, which then "fire" more neurotransmitters. Thus, a chain reaction sends substance P along a specific pathway through the brain to the sites where the sensation of pain is created. As long as substance P travels through this pathway, you feel pain.

To stop pain, substance P must be prevented from making its journey. That's what endorphins do when they stop pain. They send other neurotransmitters into the pain pathway ahead of substance P. These neurotransmitters fit the same dendrite receptors as substance P, so that when it arrives up the spinal cord, all the receptors have been filled. There is nowhere for substance P to go, and the pain stops.

The discovery of the endorphins, the key breakthrough in modern medicine's fight against chronic pain, came quite by accident. In 1973, when Avram Goldstein, a Palo Alto, California, pharmacologist, injected morphine into experimental animals, he discovered that the morphine molecules fit into receptors on the pain-pathway dendrites. Morphine did not fire the neurons, but it blocked the entry of substance P.

Why, Goldstein and other scientists asked, should the human brain created millennia ago have built-in receptors for a man-made drug developed only several decades ago? One explanation is that there are biochemicals occurring naturally in the brain that act like morphine. The search was on for the brain's own pain killers.

In 1975 a team of investigators in Aberdeen, Scotland, headed by John Hughes and Hans Kosterlitz, found the first of the brain's morphines, *enkephalin* (the word means "in the head"). Shortly thereafter, endorphin was discovered. Now the number of known endorphins has grown to about forty-five. They have been found not only in the brain, but all through the body—in the gut, the pancreas, the gonads, and the white cells.

The techniques of your pain-control program are designed to stimulate the production of endorphins, through exercise and other natural means. Many of those techniques seem bizarre because they communicate directly with the brain in special ways. But they do work. The endorphins are ten times more powerful than morphine, never lose their effectiveness as analgesic drugs do after extended use, and are safe because your body produces them naturally.

## WHAT YOU SHOULD KNOW ABOUT CHRONIC PAIN

There's a difference between acute pain, a pain that passes in seconds or weeks, and chronic pain, a pain that lasts at least six months and can go on interminably.

Acute pain serves a purpose. It's a warning signal, harsh and unmistakable, that something has gone wrong with your body. It's a message to your conscious mind to take action to remove yourself from danger. And it's a message to your unconscious mind to mobilize your body's resources to repair damage and restore your health. When you heed the warning, on the conscious level, the unconscious level, or both levels, the signal goes off. The endorphins have taken over, and the pain stops.

But the endorphins don't stop chronic pain.

Let's take a look at the nervous system to find out why. Pain begins anyplace in the body in a multitude of small nerve cells called *nociceptors,* meaning "receivers of noxious stimuli." They are thickly sprinkled over the outside of your body and throughout your insides. Their fibers—extremely fine, ultrasensitive antennae—pick up intense, potentially harmful sensations. Each is designed to pick up a specific type of pain source. Some ignore a flaming match but react to a pinprick. Some respond to a hammer blow but ignore a pinch.

As we have seen, the nociceptors transmit their reactions to the spinal cord and up to the brain, where they are converted into the sensation of pain. Their signals really travel over two routes. One, a straight, fast lane, provides the brain with instant data: the location of the pain, its intensity, and its nature—sharp, dull, throbbing, burning, or any of the other three hundred or so kinds of pain. The other, a winding, slower lane, carries the message to the brain to convert the data into the sensation of pain. The messenger is substance P, and its message is a warning signal.

Revolutionary research by two Canadian pain specialists, Dr. Patrick Wall and Dr. Ronald Melzack, indicates that a sort of gate mechanism opens to let substance P enter the spinal cord on the way to the brain and closes to keep it out.

In cases of *external injury,* the gate opens briefly to allow the warning signal to pass through, then closes rapidly to leave the injured person free of pain so all efforts can be put into fighting or fleeing whatever caused the injury. This natural protective reaction explains why we can be injured and not feel the sensation of pain return until some time later.

In cases of *internal injury*—the injury, say, of arthritis, cancer, a herniated disc, stomach cramps, and angina—the gate remains open. The reason is evident to Dr. Richard Bergland, an eminent British neurosurgeon: "Nature wants [victims of internal injury] to rest, not necessarily to take to their beds, but at least to take it easy, confident that rest will cure the pain-causing problems." However, all too frequently prolonged rest does not lead to an end of the pain, and sometimes adds to the body's problems.

The open gate explains the agonizing quality of chronic pain. "As patients with [internal] pain know well," Dr. Bergland observes, "once the gate-opening mechanism is activated, all kinds of ordinary and non-noxious stimuli are perceived by the brain as painful."

The gate may stay open long after the original noxious stimuli has been relieved. It may even open for no discernible reason. Such malfunctions account for many of the chronic pains of "unknown origin."

What exactly is the gate mechanism? It's a complex series of biochemical reactions, neurobiologists now know. Endorphins flood the gate area of the spinal cord with neurotransmitters to close the gate. If the level of endorphins falls below the level of substance P sent by the nociceptors, then the gate is open. When the mechanism that produces endorphins in the brain malfunctions, neurotransmitters that should be flowing to close the gate do not do so, and the gate remains open.

The bottom-line solution to chronic pain is to close the gate with neurotransmitters, blocking substance P with endorphins in the brain. That's what the pain-control program is all about. You'll learn ways to use your brain to stimulate the flow of endorphins.

"The gate can be adjusted by the brain to stay in closed position," Dr. Bergland comments. "The Indian fakir lying on a bed of nails has developed such control over his pain-modulating gate that he can close it at will and limit the number of pain signals that reach his brain. . . . On the other hand, the harried housewife cannot muster the brain energy to put any pressure on the brain's [endorphin-producing mechanisms] that control pain. Without that force coming from the brain, the gate remains open."

## Chronic Pain, Stress, and Depression

Dr. Bergland's harried housewife is a person under stress. Her stress, by cutting down the production of endorphins, opens the gate mechanism to substance P and keeps it open, bringing on chronic pain even though there is no physical cause. That's because "when the gate remains open," explains Dr. Bergland, "any sensation can pass through and on to the brain [as pain]. Backache, neckache, and headache are the natural consequences. . . . The pains are not imagined, they are real, but they result from the gate opening, and not from any real disease in the back, the neck, or the head."

Among the therapies of the pain-control program are total relaxation techniques that significantly reduce or eliminate the effects of stress.

Depression also opens the gate to chronic pain. All depression probably has roots in both sad external events—the loss of a job, the death of a loved one, or a divorce—and changes in the body's neurochemistry. Even depressions which are mild and so small they aren't recognized can bring on increased pain—especially in the head, neck, and back. In some of these cases, patients don't feel consciously depressed but report sleep and appetite disturbance, loss of energy and motivation, and chronic pain.

In your pain-control program, the use of nutrient supplements fights depression, while the other techniques restore high endorphin levels. All together, they work to relieve depression and close the gate on pain.

---

**3**

---

# The Old Hope and the New

---

Of the millions of Americans who seek the help of a doctor, four out of five hope to find a way of ending pain.

Traditional medicine, with earnest intent, skill, and state-of-the-art expertise, has made, and still makes, heroic efforts to ease each patient's discomfort. Its tools are mainly pain-related drugs—drugs to assuage pain, inflammation, swelling, depression, and anxiety—and surgery—from implants to nerve destruction.

These are the tools that created the old hope. While they work for some people, they don't work for all. And many people prefer not to use potentially-addicting drugs or to undergo surgery.

## TRADITIONAL TREATMENT OF THE MOST COMMON TYPES OF CHRONIC PAIN

The U. S. Department of Health and Human Services has assessed the traditional treatments for each of the six major categories of chronic pain: arthritic, cancer, headache, lower back, neurogenic (damaged nerve), and psychogenic (pain with no physical cause). Chances are that your chronic pain falls into one of these categories, and you may be undergoing one or more of the following treatments right now. Knowing what they can and can't do will help you, with the advice of your physician, to choose between traditional techniques that care for chronic pain and the new pain-control therapy.

*Arthritic pain.* Arthritis, an affliction of the joints, manifests itself in two common forms. Rheumatoid arthritis is an inflammation—a condition of redness and swelling accompanied by heat and pain—of the soft tissue around the joints. Osteoarthritis is a degeneration of the bone and cartilage associated with the joints; with symptoms akin to those of rheumatoid arthritis, it typically affects the fingers and may spread to the hips or spine.

Traditional methods are most effective on arthritis pain when the disease is treated early. Drugs are the major ingredient in traditional treatment. "The most widely used. . .and important drug," according to a panel of pain-control experts, is aspirin. Almost as widely prescribed are steroid drugs—pharmaceuticals that are synthetic near-counterparts of the body's own anti-inflammatory agents manufactured in the adrenal glands. There are also non-steroid anti-inflammatory drugs like indomethacin and ibuprofen. All drugs, even aspirin, have the risk of serious adverse side effects. For example, extended use of steroids induces damage to the immune system and consequent lowered resistance to infection. Hemorrhaging is not uncommon, and habitual steroid users are usually characterized by facial puffiness—the "steroid moonface."

Exercise is part of the traditional as well as of the new therapy, and seems to be the key to the successful treatment of arthritis pain. Exercise in warm water is especially effective: the heated liquid is relaxing, and the water buoys up the body against the force of gravity, allowing exercise to be taken with little exertion. If arthritis is not advanced, a modest program of aspirin and other anti-inflammatory drugs, combined with exercise, can restore the joints to full function and help ward off future degeneration. Warm or cold compresses provide additional pain relief.

When arthritis is in its advanced stages, the traditional treatment sometimes falls back on surgery. A diseased joint, in which tissue has been destroyed, is replaced on the operating table with an artificial joint. A prime example of this generally successful type of operation is the total hip replacement. But since all major surgery carries risks, including chronic post-operative pain, it is always best to treat arthritis early.

*Cancer pain.* The intolerable agony of cancer can result from the pressure of a growing tumor, from the tumor's destruction of bone and tissue, from its invasion of cells and organs, and from its attacks on the carriers of pain itself, the nerves. Sadly, the standard therapies for inoperable cancers, radiation and chemotherapy, can grossly intensify the pain. "These treatments," explains the National Institute of Health, "can cause fluid accumulation and swelling (edema), irritate or destroy healthy tissue. . . , and possibly sensitize nerve endings [to pain]."

*Headache pain.* The two most common forms are tension headache and migraine headache. Tension headache, one of the stress-related diseases epidemic in modern civilization, erupts from continued contractions of the muscles of the head and neck. Migraine, the most infamous member of a group of vascular headaches, explodes when there are unexpected variations of blood pressure in the vessels supplying the brain. The intense throbbing pain on one side of the head characteristic of migraine is the result of the abrupt "swing-swangs" of blood pressure during the course of the headache.

Both types of headache pain are treated by traditional medicine with therapeutic drugs. They provide some temporary relief for some victims of tension headaches. However, they are useful to some migraine sufferers only when taken at the onset of the pain, or even before, when the aura—a dazzling display of zigzagging lights—first appears. Besides other drugs, traditional medicine offers temporary alleviation with hot or cold compresses.

*Lower back pain.* To relieve the muscle tension of lower back pain, muscle-relaxant tranquilizers and bed rest are usually prescribed. While at first this treatment is rated effective to very effective, over the long run it is ineffective. Protracted use of muscle-relaxants worsens the condition, increasing pain and causing depression. Extended bed rest is an unsatisfactory solution both physically—muscles waste away from disuse—and psychologically—the bed becomes a prison.

In some stubborn cases, a traditional doctor may prescribe a complete examination of the body's network of nerves, highlighted by a myelogram, an X ray of the spinal cord. The object is to discover whether there is painful pressure on the spinal cord or its sensitive nerves, such as that caused by a herniated disk. The disks separate the body units of the spinal cord, the vertebrae; when a disk is herniated, it has been broken apart and squeezed into the spinal canal by the pair of vertebrae around it. If a herniated disk is found, it is treated by surgery. But hospital records show that neither a myelogram nor surgery is foolproof.

Some doctors, in transition to the new therapy of chronic pain, see lower back pain as a disease of Western civilization. It is caused, they believe, by a combination of bad posture, worsened by a bulging belly, and a sedentary life. Their approach to long-term help is to prescribe mild analgesics, including aspirin, plus a weight-control program and exercises. It's a commendable step toward a total pain-control program.

*Neurogenic pain.* This pain arises from damage to the central nervous system, made up of the brain and spinal cord, or the peripheral nervous system, which branches out from the spinal cord to the various parts of the body. The three most common neurogenic pains are those of tic, shingles, and phantom-limb pain.

Tic (trigeminal neuralgia) is a recurrent, stabbing pain in the facial area. Because it occurs more frequently among the old than among the young, it is suspected that it is caused by a degeneration of the nervous system, inducing excessive activity (firing) of brain cells. However, any kind of damage to the nervous system can produce the same symptoms at any age. Traditional treatment of tic is based mainly on drugs designed to quiet epileptic seizures, which are also associated with excessive firing of the brain cells. Such antiepileptic drugs (Tegretol, generic name carbamazepine, is an example) are effective in as short a time as twenty-four to seventy-two hours, but they produce adverse side effects. Among over-sixties, the major target of this disease, side effects are likely to be intensified. Another treatment for tic is surgical: a small sponge is inserted between blood vessels and the nerves that supply sensory fibers to the face to reduce pressure on the nerves.

Shingles (herpes zoster) is a neuralgia induced by a virus related to the herpes viruses that cause common cold sores and sexually transmitted herpes (herpes simplex I and II). It produces an extraordinary searing pain. Shingles is treated with the same type of drugs that are prescribed for tic, bringing the same advantages and drawbacks.

Phantom pain is felt in a limb that has been lost or paralyzed. Combinations of anti-depressant drugs and mild narcotic analgesics are sometimes effective, but side effects can be hazardous, and the narcotic analgesics can be habit-forming.

*Psychogenic pain.* This is a category of pain for which no physical cause can be found. But this doesn't mean that it's "all in the mind," in the sense that it doesn't exist. If you feel chronic pain, the chances are that the pain is real, not hallucinated or imagined. Traditional medicine has been baffled by psychogenic pain and has found no reliable way to treat it.

A possible explanation for this strange disease, based on the discoveries of the new pain therapists, is that the neurotransmitters that control the pain system are in imbalance. That consideration has paved the way to a successful therapy: the stimulation of greater production of endorphins. Treatment of psychogenic pain is one outstanding example of the success of the new therapy, bringing pain sufferers new hope.

## OLD AND NEW HOPES

*The old hope for Maria Fichter was drugs.*

Her pain had started shortly after a hysterectomy. Maria says, "I was just twenty-seven. I thought when you get old and creaky, that's when you start to hurt. I thought it could never happen to me."

She described her pain as "a throbbing, pulsating thing. I can feel it in my temple on the left side. I can hear it in my ears. My eyes are very sensitive to light. In bright lights I feel a tremendous pressure on my eyes." At age forty she had lived with that pain almost every day for thirteen years, until it become "utterly unbearable."

Diagnosis: Migraine, among the most vicious of headaches.

Treatment: Fiorinal with codeine, a powerful sedative/narcotic, and Levo-Dromoran, a potent narcotic analgesic.

But the migraines multiplied in frequency and intensity. Sometimes they lasted for three days running. Daily migraines sometimes went on for hours. Often the migraines would come in clusters, one after another like repeated hammer blows. "I would stagger on the street, and the neighbors would think I was drunk." Between migraines she lived in fear of those horrible headaches striking again, and of a "big one" that might culminate in stroke.

The narcotic drugs and tranquilizers Maria took to relieve her pain and anxieties became another problem. "They made me dopey, so I drank black coffee to pep me up, but then it would let me down—hard. So I took pep pills. I was 'up' and 'down' like a yoyo." When Maria realized that her hope for relief through drugs was gone, that she might have to live the rest of her life in pain without hope of healing, her depression deepened. "I thought, What's the use? I thought of suicide."

*The new hope* came to Maria Fichter when she was hooked to a biofeedback machine that measured the temperature of her hands and displayed the result for her. Biofeedback is a technique for watching your body (your *bio*logical being) telling you how it responds to your commands and actions (providing you with *feedback*). Maria willed the temperature of her hands to rise, and she saw the numbers go up and up on the machine's thermometric digital printout. Biofeedback gave her proof that she could bring about positive changes in her body. And as Maria's hands grew warmer and warmer, the pain in her head grew less and less.

"Your migraine is caused by blood vessels in your head quickly tightening and then swelling," she was told by her new pain-control specialist. "When you will your hands to get warmer, you make the blood vessels in your hands swell. You interrupt the constriction of blood vessels in your head, and that aborts your headache." Said the astonished Maria, "That was the greatest day of my life. I—can you imagine it—I could just will my pain away."

Maria's total pain-control program does not include narcotic analgesics and sedative drugs. In fact, two months of the new "pain capsule" regimen that was part of Maria's program freed her from the drugs that had done her no good and, she says, had increased her pain and suffering. Today, Maria has an occasional migraine, but it's mild; it passes in twenty minutes or so, and leaves only a light residue of pain.

*The old hope for Linda Fallon was surgery.*

"I was terrified of surgery, the idea of being cut up and then sewed together again. . . . Well, I didn't want to think about it."

But what else was she to do? Three years earlier she had been in a car accident, and ever since then she had been in indescribable pain. "The doctors said I had a crushed nerve in my leg. It was so painful that putting on my panties was a horrible experience. My neck, my back, my shoulders, all hurt so. When I reached up to take a can from the shelf, the pain was like a red-hot knife cutting through me.

"Drugs helped some, but just some. I had a four-year-old; I had a husband. I had to take care of them, but I couldn't. I felt my family was going to fall apart, my husband would leave me, my kid grow up to hate me. I felt guilty. It would all be my fault if I didn't have the operation."

There are two kinds of pain surgery: surgery that treats the cause of pain, and surgery that cuts the nerves which carry pain. The first type includes the removal of a tumor, the repair of a herniated disk, and bypass surgery to reduce the pain of angina. Surgery that treats the cause of pain is commonly prescribed, has a high safety rating, and is by and large effective. Still, no surgery is successful for everybody; all surgery is hazardous and carries the risk of chronic postoperative pain for some people.

Linda Fallon underwent the other type of pain surgery, which cuts the nerves that transmit pain. Her doctor severed certain nerves in her spinal column which carried the message of pain from her leg to her brain. Neurosurgeons have achieved some excellent results with this technique, even in difficult brain and upper spinal cord surgery.

But nerve-severing surgery carries a burden of possible dangers. It may eliminate not only pain, but other sensations as well—warmth, coolness, and taste, for example, It may—and surgeons can't predict this outcome in individual cases—become a source of new pain. The most disheartening result is that the magic release from pain may not last long. After six months to a year, the pain may return for some patients, and Linda Fallon was one of those.

"At first I felt as though I was in heaven," she says. "But after a while I felt numb. I don't know how to tell people this, but the numbness was as bad as the pain. A horrible sensation. And then the pain came back." For Linda, the failure of surgery meant the end of hope. "I didn't know where to go, what to do. I couldn't deal with it anymore."

*The new hope* came to Linda Fallon with a therapy "as far apart from surgery as you can imagine." It was guided imagery—the movies of the mind. In a state of deep relaxation, she projected a short fantasy in her mind.

*Linda imagined that her hand pulled out the red-hot knife that caused her pain.*

The image of the knife communicated with that part of her brain that controls endorphins, and a flood of endorphins overwhelmed her pain. She imagined that the knife came out, and her pain went away. Guided imagery was integrated with many other new therapies in Linda's total pain-control program.

Linda Fallon is almost free of pain. She's also free of guilt and her overriding fear of her family's breaking up.

*The old hope for Willis Hoskinson was electrodes implanted in his brain.*

Willis was an arthritic. The crippling disease was in his back, in his hands, and in his legs. "My back hurt so much I couldn't sit in a chair. My fingers were so swollen and stiff and painful I couldn't hold a pen to write a letter. I couldn't walk," this sixty-six-year-old former athlete said. What hurt Willis most was that he couldn't play with his grandchildren.

When his doctor told him about implanting electrodes in his brain, Willis eagerly agreed to the operation. The doctor explained that certain areas in the brain can alleviate pain when they're stimulated electrically. Tiny electrodes, terminals for an electric current, are placed surgically into these areas. The source of the electric current is a portable device outside the body, regulated by the patient. When the patient is in need of pain relief, he simply twists a dial.

Electrical brain stimulation has a high success rate. In tests conducted at Stanford University in California, two out of three patients received significant pain relief from this treatment, though followup studies show that its effect decreases over time. There are risks, of course, in brain surgery. For Willis, though, his disease was so severe that nothing else could be done for him. This was his last resort.

The operation went perfectly. "That little device was a godsend," Willis said. "I just turned it on the right voltage, and it was like turning off the pain." He could play with his grandchildren again.

But not for long. For Willis, repeated stimulation progressively decreased effectiveness, and in several months, even at the highest voltage, the pain-killing power of the electrodes was minimal. "I felt there was no hope anymore."

*The new hope* came to Willis Hoskinson through his total pain-control program, which featured exercises and self-hypnosis. The exercises helped loosen his rigid joints. Hypnotic suggestion opened his unconscious brain to his commands to end pain, initiating a flow of pain-killing endorphins. The total pain-control program did not cure Willis's arthritis—in the present stage of our knowledge, it is an irreversible disease—but it reduced his pain to a steady level he can cope with.

*The old hope for Felix Schramm was "nerve blocks."*

Confined to a wheelchair at twenty-six after his car was totaled by a truck jumping the divider on a freeway, Felix suffered so much, so constantly, that he cried and screamed at night.

Diagnosis: Musculoskeletal pain (pain arising from abnormal pressure of muscles and bone on adjacent nerves).

Treatment: Nerve blocks.

This treatment, in essence, temporarily blocks pain impulses from the injured area from reaching the brain with the injection of a local anesthetic. When your dentist gives you Novocaine or a related drug, he or she is treating your pain-to-come with nerve blocks. Nerve blocks supply instant and, to many chronic-pain sufferers, what seems to be, "miraculous relief." The effect endures for a considerable time after the local anesthetic has worn off, and repeated nerve blocks can supply pain relief lasting up to years.

Nerve blocks are the outstanding achievements of traditional medicine's pain therapy. Their results are consistently good to excellent. But nerve blocks have drawbacks. When you're an outpatient this treatment means returning to the clinic for injections possibly every day. Moreover, the relief does not treat the cause of pain, just as your dentist's Novocaine does not treat your rotting tooth, so nerve blocks cannot end the pain. The pain can develop a tolerance for the anesthetic and return in a more terrible form than ever.

As it did to Felix Schramm.

*The new hope* came to Felix when he learned that at modern pain-control centers nerve blocks are used as a transition to the new therapies that hold out hope of permanent relief. He was put on a total pain-relief program that emphasized physical therapy, exercise, and sound nutrition in addition to other nonsurgical pain-control treatments. His muscles and bones strengthened, pressure on his nerves lessened, and his pain diminished. Felix is out of the wheelchair and claims to have achieved 95 percent relief of pain.

*The old hope for Clive Parker was psychotherapy for a pain no one could understand.*

Clive's pain had come out of the blue—no accident, no illness. Clive Parker had always eaten right, exercised right, lived right, and yet he was afflicted with a terrifying pain syndrome. Diffuse pain in his back, neck, and shoulder radiated to his arms, legs, and buttocks. X rays, CAT scans, and electromyographs (EMG's) revealed no source of pain in his body, brain, or nerves.

Diagnosis: Psychosomatic pain, the type characterized by doctors as being "all in the head."

Treatment: Psychotherapy.

It helped. It helped soften the stress of the pain experience. It helped dispel some of the depression of being a pain victim, depression which only adds to the suffering. It helped prevent Clive from becoming that sad person whose life revolves around his pain. But it didn't help his pain.

It couldn't help, because his pain had been misdiagnosed. Clive's doctors, in their traditional approach, had eliminated one test that has become a standard procedure of the new pain-control specialists in cases of "pain of unknown origin." That test is a ther-mogram, a picture of the heat patterns of the body from which doctors can identify points whose temperatures are abnormally high. These points have been associated with tender spots in the body's soft tissue, and when touched they appear to trigger pain at distant sites in the body.

*The new hope* came to Clive Parker when he was shown his thermogram, which revealed that his pain was not in his head, but real, and in many parts of his body. "I knew I wasn't nuts! What a relief! Pure, absolutely pure joy!" His hope rose when he was told that his disease, myofascial pain syndrome, was not uncommon, though medicine had not come up with a definite explanation for this mysterious condition.

Clive began to receive intermittent relief from trigger point therapy, injections of long-lasting local anesthetics at the tender spots that trigger pain. He enthusiastically embraced a total pain-control program as an outpatient. The program prescribed for Clive was much like your pain-control program will be, except that it was supplemented by trigger-point injections administered by his doctor. Several months after starting the program, Clive esti-mated that he enjoyed about 90 percent pain relief, and shortly afterwards that figure reached a permanent 100 percent.

These are the encouraging results of the new pain-control ther-apies, used alongside or instead of traditional methods. Combining the decades of experience of traditional doctors with the new wave of laboratory and clinical research on pain, pioneers in new pain-control therapy have succeeded in recognizing the true nature of chronic pain and the best techniques for treating it. Because of these breakthroughs, you will never again have to give up hope of escape from pain.

## TOTAL BENEFITS OF NEW PAIN-CONTROL THERAPIES

In the following chapters you will become acquainted with the new therapies that provide the new hope:

- exercises
- total relaxation techniques
- autogenics and self-hypnosis
- pain-control imagery
- nutrients to help control pain-related depression
- a nutritious diet to help build a sound defense against pain
- effortless drug withdrawal
- a new attitude toward yourself and your pain

It is important to think of your pain-control program as a total package in which every part works together. You should not treat it like a smorgasbord from which you can pick and choose treatments. Chronic pain is like a fire with many fuels. Unless all the fuels are eliminated, the fire won't go out. Each chapter from four to eleven addresses one of the fuels of chronic pain. Within some chapters, alternative methods are given, but it is important to utilize techniques from every chapter. In that way, you achieve the total benefits of your pain-control program.

In addition to offering relief from pain, as the traditional treatments do, the new pain-control therapies improve your health overall. Better health, in turn, leads to feeling better about yourself and to gaining even more strength to fight pain.

For instance, exercise is a major part of the new therapy because it stimulates the production of endorphins, fights stress by relaxing tense muscles, and relieves depression by triggering the flow of feel-good substances in the brain. At the same time, any good fitness program has the following well-established advantages. You increase muscular strength and flexibility. You help ward off heart attack and other degenerative diseases. You increase your blood supply, bringing ample quantities of precious oxygen, nutrients, and your own body's medicinals to every cell of your body. You reverse joint stiffness. Your stamina rises, as do your endurance and strength. You find yourself capable of physical feats you wouldn't have dared before you began to exercise. All this, in addition to helping relieve your pain.

Similarly, a pain-control diet not only contains large amounts of the nutrients that fight pain and depression, it is essentially a good-health diet, of the type approved by the American Medical

Association for everybody. Not only do you feel better emotionally, but this diet puts you on the road to good physical health. It helps slim you down and keep you slim. It fights heart attack, cardiovascular diseases, and high blood pressure. It's a foe of diabetes, gout, diverticulosis (a disorder of the large bowel), and constipation. It combats gallstones and cataracts. It strengthens your immune system and helps ward off infection. It boosts your energy, and it helps sharpen your brain. You feel better all over.

Most importantly, the new chronic-pain therapies help lift your emotions. The worst reaction to pain that you can have is to give up hope. Despair leads to depression, and depression to more pain. Every part of your pain-control program, from total relaxation techniques to autogenics, will show you that you have the resources to beat your pain. With the supervision of your physician, you can control what you recently thought was controlling you.

# PART TWO

# YOUR
# CHRONIC-PAIN-CONTROL
# PROGRAM

# 4

# Pain-Control Exercises
# Anyone Can Do

Your body in motion—regularly, vigorously—is a potent ther-apy for pain; in the opinion of some chronic-pain specialists, it is perhaps the most potent. Simple exercises that anyone can do, including some that can be done anywhere, can reap enormous benefits.

Endorphins, the brain's own painkillers, flow more freely. Stress, that vicious intensifier of pain, is subdued. Your body's general overall health, nature's basic defense against chronic pain, is lifted. You feel *good* when you exercise.

It's been years since I've felt any pain in my lower back, but I continue to exercise, for I know it's as strong a preventive against pain as it is a therapeutic. Exercise can help you, no matter what kind of chronic pain you suffer, as it helped and continues to help me to freedom from chronic pain and to fitness and health. Exercise for life—for the sake of your life.

If you're like most Americans, exercise has little or no part in your life. Despite the swelling interest in fitness, it is estimated by pain-control specialists that only about four adult Americans in one hundred exercise sufficiently to have a positive influence on chronic pain.

As a chronic-pain sufferer fearful of aggravating your pain by added physical activity, you may approach exercise with apprehension. And, if you're not an exerciser, what you feared usually occurs when you begin to exercise, when the initial impact of exertion on little-used muscles induces soreness and increases discomfort. That's why the exercise program recommended here has been designed to ease you gently into fitness—and painlessness.

## WHAT WE'VE LEARNED ABOUT PAIN-CONTROL EXERCISES AT THE PAIN ALLEVIATION CENTER

Take the case of Vera Alden. About thirty-five, married, with two teenage sons, she had suffered intense headache and neck pains for nearly three years after a car accident. She had been put on narcotic analgesics to which she had built a tolerance—"I needed more and more but felt less and less relief"—and was finally placed in traction. It failed.

Extremely sensitive to touch, she was unable to hold a job, do household chores, or make love. Her marriage, her relations with her sons, and her self-esteem were coming apart. Her consistently nonsuccessful response to medical treatment forced her into believing, as one doctor had concluded, that it was, indeed,[11] all in her head." She felt hopeless and helpless, and that magnified her pain.

Referred to us, she was introduced for the first time to physical therapy, along with a total pain-control program that included biofeedback and other deep relaxation techniques. At the nation's advanced pain-control centers, physical therapy to treat chronic pain is administered through exercises with the aid of machines. It provided Vera, says, with "immediate short-term relief."

She was then encouraged to make exercise without mechanical help a part of her life away from the center. Her outpatient exercise program, very much like the one outlined in this chapter, fortified with the other techniques of the new pain-control therapy, turned short-term relief into long-term relief.

Vera regards her away-from-the-center exercise program as the turning point of her life. Virtually free of pain, she has integrated the broken pieces of her life, is a loving and loved wife and mother, and is back at her job. Life for her is as it was before the accident, she says, except for the one new element that continues to add to her well-being: exercise.

The type of at-home exercises that helped Vera and many other outpatients, male and female, appear in this chapter. (They are not a substitute for physical therapy; and you should consult the physician supervising your pain-control therapy about your need for that kind of therapy.) While the exercises described in this chapter—your pain-control exercises—do help to relieve some *specific* kinds of pain, especially those related to the musculoskeletal system, the thrust of the regimen is to reduce chronic pain of every kind wherever it occurs.

In this chapter, you'll also find pain-relieving exercises that are easy to do in your home and some you can do away from home. You'll discover how they work. You'll also discover what their benefits are, not only for the alleviation of your pain, but for overall mental and physical well-being. You'll be provided with easy-to-follow instructions, so you can get going at once.

Try to think of these exercises as the start of an exciting new adventure with your body. For, from the simple exercises with which you begin, you can reach out to new, and forgotten, joys of your body in motion: walking, jogging, running, dancing, swimming—added pleasures in your life without pain.

## HOW PAIN-CONTROL EXERCISES WORK

The practice of rubbing a hurt region of the body to ease the pain is as old as humankind. Kissing away the pain of a child's bruises is as ancient as motherhood. Whole systems of muscular manipulation to ease pain have flourished throughout civilized times, most notably the Hindu discipline of yoga. Muscles have responded for millennia to massaging hands that smooth away pain. In the heat of battle, in the hunt, in sex, in the fierce rivalry of athletes in competition, churning muscles have always slammed the door on pain.

Built into our beings, it now appears, is a mechanism that connects body parts in motion—vigorous, high-energy motion—with the release of endorphins. At the same time, certain substances in the brain—mainly the neurotransmitters norepinephrine (NE) and dopamine (DA)—give you a can't-lose feeling of certainty and self-confidence, the very opposite of the helplessness and hopelessness of chronic pain. The "runner's high" may well be a sort of intoxication brought on by those substances. The total syndrome induced by exercise fights not only pain in all parts of the body, but also depression, which adversely affects functions throughout the body.

At the same time, muscles in motion are acting to relieve local pain. In chronic pain, some pain-control specialists surmise, muscles have "frozen" into states of tension. Contracted and rigid, they produce certain biochemicals, the kinins, which continually send out pain signals. Unfreezing the muscles into fluidity through exercise cuts off the flow of the kinins, ending their pain signals. Exercise also heightens the blood flow to the affected regions, carrying a bounty of warmth, nourishment, and oxygen—a natural therapeutic for pain.

Acting at the pain source and throughout the body, exercise works to help you win your battle against pain.

# GETTING MENTALLY PREPARED TO EXERCISE

If you're like many of my patients, you may still not be convinced that exercise is right for you. Doctors may have told you, "If it hurts, don't do it." Your common sense affirms that advice. But well-intentioned and valid as it is in some situations for some kinds of acute pain, that advice could severely retard, or even prevent, your recovery from chronic pain.

Exercise is necessary and it's doable. If your mind says no to exercise, it's time you changed it. Construct a new positive attitude to exercise with these clinically proven facts.

- *When you start to exercise, hurt does not necessarily mean harm.* Yes, you will hurt at first. But far from being a sign of harm, it's a sign that something good is happening to you. Your muscles, which have been inactive for a long time, are coming back to life.
- *When you continue to exercise, you can prevent yourself from hurting.* You do this by establishing your "hurt threshold": the amount of exercise you can do before you begin to hurt. If, for example, you begin to hurt, which means that you hurt more than you usually do, after three minutes of walking, then three minutes is your hurt threshold. Stay below that threshold, and you won't hurt.

  Find your hurt threshold for each of the recommended exercises in this chapter by observing, over the course of a few days or a week or so, how many times you can repeat each one before you begin to hurt. Keep a day-by-day record (your hurt threshold is likely to fluctuate) and settle on the lowest value. If for example, the numbers run 2, 2, 3, 2, 4, 3, 2, select 2.
- *When you exercise regularly, you will feel so good that you will want to exercise more and more.* And you should. But don't overdo it.

Start your recommended program of exercise at two thirds of your hurt threshold (say, six repetitions of the exercise instead of nine), then increase repetitions by one every few days. A wonderful thing will then happen to you, as it does to many patients. When you reach your hurt threshold of nine, in this case, you won't hurt. The exercise will actually raise your hurt threshold.

Continue to increase your repetitions to find your new hurt threshold. Cut back again to two thirds of it, then increase the repetitions—and once again you may find that you have raised your hurt threshold. By elevating your hurt threshold bit by bit, you'll soon be able to perform all the repetitions required by the recommended exercise program—without hurting.

**Caution:** The exercise program will make you feel so good that you may be tempted to rush your development and increase the number of repetitions too much, too soon. Then you *will* hurt for days, or even weeks. But because the exercise program proves so beneficial to you, you'll be champing at the bit to get back to it, and, as soon as you feel a little better, you do. But, once more, you overdo. Once more, the hurt. Once more, the return to the program. Once more, the overdo. Once more, the hurt. Once more, the return to the program. And on and on and on. You're trapped in "the chronic-pain exercise cycle."

Avoid it by reaching your maximum pain threshold bit by bit. When you reach that threshold, you'll be able to perform all the required repetitions of the following exercises without hurting. These exercises can help you to a pain-free life.

---

### INSTRUCTIONS FOR PERFORMING YOUR PAIN-CONTROL EXERCISES

Before starting this exercise program, or any such program, consult the physician supervising your pain-control program.

#### Your Basic Exercises

See page 39 for suggested timetable.

---

## Get-Going Exercises

These are simple stretching exercises to perform in bed before you get up in the morning. They are a warmup for your day's activities, stretching and limbering up your muscles and gently speeding the actions of your heart and lungs for the day's exertions. They also reduce the possibility of strain when you perform other exercises. Most important: They stimulate the flow of endorphins.

In the following exercises, s-t-r-e-t-c-h s-l-o-w-l-y. Don't strain. Don't bounce. S-t-r-e-t-c-h more and more, very gradually, until you feel a slight pull. Hold for 30 seconds. Then try to stretch a *little* more. Hold for another 30 seconds. You'll get a feeling of warmth (your blood is stirring) and relaxation (your tight muscles are loosening up).

1. Start with your feet (remember, you're in bed). Lying on your back, bend your knees. Grasp your left foot in both hands, and stretch it up gently for 15 seconds, then down for 15 seconds. Repeat with your right foot.

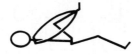

2. Keeping your knees bent, bring your left knee to your chest in 15 to 30 seconds, in the meantime straightening your right knee on your bed. Repeat, bringing your right knee to your chest and straightening your left knee. Bring both your knees to your chest for 30 seconds. This exercise stretches lower back muscles.

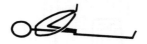

**41**

3. Turn over and lie flat on your stomach for 30 seconds. Prop yourself up on your elbows and hold your chin in your hands for 60 seconds. This exercise stretches abdominal and hip muscles, as well as some of the spinal ligaments.

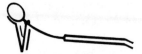

4. Sit up and hang your legs over the side of your bed, placing your feet on the floor. Let your chest fall slowly to your knees while your arms hang down to the floor. Take 30 seconds to perform this. This exercise stretches back muscles and relaxes the muscles of arms and shoulders.

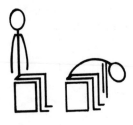

5. Sit on the edge of your bed in the starting position of exercise 4. Stretch your neck muscles by looking all the way to your left for 30 seconds (you'll feel a gentle pull, but don't

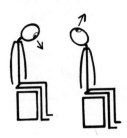

strain), then to your right for 30 seconds. Let your chin fall gently to your chest and permit the weight of your head to stretch the back of your neck for 30 seconds. Let your head fall back gently and look at the ceiling for 30 seconds. (If this action produces pain, you may first want to support your head with your hands.)

## Keep-Going Exercises

"Keep-Going" means getting through the day with less strain and pain, and less depression than you have had. This general exercise program for just about anyone has three objectives: to increase strength, to increase flexibility, and to increase cardiovascular endurance. Reaching all three of these objectives will help to reduce your pain.

## Exercises to increase strength in all major muscle groups

1. *Calf raises.* Using a wall for balance, rise on the balls of your feet as far as possible, then slowly return your heels to the ground. (The best way to perform this exercise is barefoot or in socks or slippers.) Repeat 10 times. As your strength improves, increase to 15 times, adding one repetition every few days.

   As your flexibility improves through the stretching program you will perform following these strengthening exercises, place the balls of your feet on a step, with your heels extended over the edge. Let your heels drop below the level of the balls of your feet, then raise your heels as far as possible. Repeat 15 times. (Or instead of using a step, use a sturdy two-inch-thick board fastened to the floor or ground.) **Caution**: Take care not to slip while performing this exercise.

   As your strength improves further, repeat the exercises one leg at a time, at first using your hands against a wall for support. Then, as you grow stronger, try it without support; when you're even stronger, hold weights or heavy books in your hands.

These exercises strengthen the calf muscles.

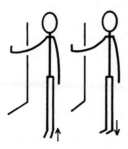

2. *Knee bends (not deep).* Standing with your feet shoulder-level apart or a little wider, feet pointing straight ahead or at a 45-degree angle outward (these positions can be varied from day to day), bend your knees until your thighs are approximately parallel to the floor. (You may have to work gradually toward this parallel position, starting with slight bends and progressively deepening them.) Repeat 10 times and progress gradually to 15 or up to 20 times.

When your strength improves significantly, perform this exercise on one leg, using a heavy piece of furniture for balance and support. Keep your back straight and erect throughout the exercise.

This exercise strengthens the quadriceps (the great thigh muscle) and develops your capability to lift packages by using your legs instead of putting all the strain on your back. You probably have been told to lift this way, but didn't have the strength to do it. This exercise supplies that strength. It also strengthens the powerful supportive muscles of the hips and buttocks.

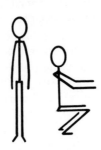

3. *Lower back muscle exercise.* Other exercise programs provide for stretching, but rarely strengthening, these muscles.

Starting position: With your knees bent, lean back over a table or low dresser, supporting yourself with your arms. Experiment until you find furniture of the height that's right for you. You'll also have to determine the proper degree of bending by trial and error.

Using your arms to help take most of the strain off your back, but also using your lower back muscles to some extent, straighten your back to an upright position. Lower yourself gently back to the starting position, using your arms for support. As your strength increases, use your arms for support less and less, and depend more and more on your back muscles. Repeat 10 times, and progress to 15 as you become stronger.

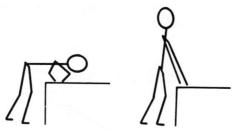

4. *Crunch sit-ups.* To strengthen abdominal muscles. Lie on the floor, a rug, or a cushion and hook your feet under a bed or other low piece of furniture with your knees bent 90 degrees and your hands at your sides. *Curl* your body toward your knees, starting with your chin, then following with your shoulders, and so on. As you do this, think of *crunching* your lower ribs toward your hips. Your head and shoulders will curl up, but not your lower back, which you should not lift off the floor. Repeat 10 times, progressing to 15.

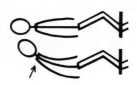

As your strength increases, cross your arms over your chest so they act as weights. When you're able to lift those weights with ease, place them behind your head. That's more difficult, but it will give you added strength.

5. *Easy push-ups.* Lie face down on a mat or carpeted floor, placing both your palms on the floor directly under your shoulders. Press up, using your knees as a fulcrum (see illustration). Repeat 10 times, progressing to 15 as your strength increases. As it increases further, you can graduate to regular push-ups, without using your knees as a fulcrum. As your flexibility increases, you might try pushing up between two telephone books or other books of equal thickness. This will enable you to stretch your pectoral (chest) muscles before pushing up. Basically, this exercise strengthens arm, shoulder, and chest muscles. It also helps take some pressure off your back as you use your arms to get in and out of cars, get up from chairs, and so forth.

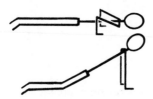

6. *Easy chin-ups.* Kneel on a carpeted floor by an open door. Grip the knobs on each side of the door with each hand. Extend your arms, keeping your back straight. Your knees should be close to the door, but your back should be leaning away from it at about a 45-degree angle. Slowly pull yourself toward the door to an upright position. (If you suffer from dizzy spells, make sure you don't perform this exercise while you are alone.) This is a particularly effective exercise for strengthening upper back, shoulder, and arm muscles, perfectly complementing the preceding exercise. Repeat 10 times; progress to 15 as your strength increases.

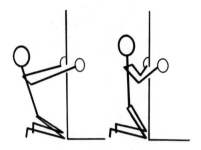

7. *Neck exercise.* Place your palms on your forehead and press them backward as you press forward with your head to resist the hand pressure. Time: 6 seconds. Place your palms against the back of your head and press back on them with your head. Time: 6 seconds. Repeat the exercise on the left and right sides of your head for 6 seconds each. Your neck muscles resist the palm pressure, thereby becoming strengthened.

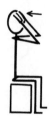

*Exercises to increase flexibility.* These stretch exercises are most effective when performed immediately after the *exercises to increase strength.*

1. *Calf stretch.* Place your hands against a wall, your left leg back with knee locked, right leg forward, knee bent for support. Stretch your left calf muscle gently for 15 to 30 seconds, then stretch slightly harder for another 15 to 30 seconds. Reverse legs and repeat.

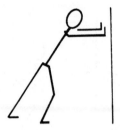

2. *Thigh stretch.* Stand on your right leg, using a wall or sturdy furniture for support. Grasp your left ankle with your left hand behind your back and pull gently, stretching your thigh. Hold for 30 seconds. Repeat on other side.

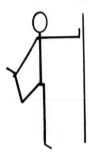

3. *Back stretch.* Repeat *get-going exercise 2.*
4. *Back extension stretch.* These are probably the most misunderstood of all exercises, even by many physicians. These doctors tell their back patients to do flexion exercises (like *exercise to increase flexibility 3* and *exercise to increase strength 4*) but to avoid all extension or hyperextension exercises.

But those exercises are very effective in the treatment of back problems. Recommended by the Canadian physical therapist Robin McKenzie, who claims that they may even help reduce the pressure of herniated disk against spinal nerves, they have produced excellent results for lower back patients at the Pain Alleviation Center. Some of those patients suffered from disk herniation, which was documented by X rays, CAT scans, and other tests.

Here is a simple back extension exercise. Lie on your stomach for a few seconds to a few minutes. Prop yourself up on your elbows, as in *get-going exercise 3,* for a few seconds to a few minutes. As your flexibility increases, press your back further upward with your hands and forearms. Keep the pressing time brief. Repeat 10 times.

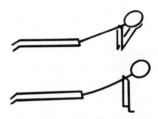

5. *Chest stretch.* Stand in a doorway, your hands at either side at shoulder height, touching the sides of the doorway. Gently step forward, leaving your hands on the doorway, until you feel a slight pull on your chest muscles. Hold for 30 seconds.

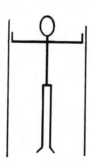

6. *Upper back stretch.* Stretch your left arm in front of your body and bring it across your chest. Hook your right arm under

your left elbow and pull it gently across your body to your right side. Feel the gentle stretch for 30 seconds, reverse arms, and repeat.

7. Repeat *get-going exercise 5.*

*Exercises to increase cardiovascular endurance (aerobic exercises).* These exercises are defined as those that cause the heart rate to reach 60 to 80 percent of maximum, sustained for 20 to 30 minutes, 3 or more times a week. They can produce not only cardiovascular conditioning, but also probably stimulate the flow of endorphins in the central nervous system. They are especially valuable to chronic-pain sufferers because they are not strenuous or exhausting. Aerobic exercises include walking, stationary bicycling or actual bicycling, swimming, and dancing. Starting with gentle exercises like these, many back patients can graduate to such strenuous exercises as jogging, running, and tennis.

Before you begin an aerobic exercise program, the physician supervising your pain-control program will in all likelihood prescribe a stress test, in addition to a general physical, to determine the state of your cardiovascular health. Cardiovascular refers to the blood vessels connected with the heart. Should your test results indicate that you are a candidate for aerobic exercises, we recommend that you start with walking.

Determine your hurt threshold (see page 39) and start at a number that is about two thirds of it. If, for example, your hurt threshold is 6 minutes of walking, start with 4 minutes each day. Then extend your walking time each day by 30 seconds to a minute. When you've reached 6 minutes, you'll be pleasantly surprised to find that you feel no pain. Your walking will create a new hurt threshold, perhaps at 7 or 10 minutes. Continue to extend the pain threshold by adding 30 seconds' to a minute's walking time until you can walk for 20 minutes without interruption. Then check with your supervising physician to determine whether you're ready for longer walks or other types of aerobic exercises.

## APPLYING YOUR BASIC EXERCISES TO SPECIFIC PAINS

*For lower back pain,* emphasize *exercises to increase flexibility 3 and 4* and *exercises to increase strength 2, 3, and 4.* Repeat these exercises twice, then, after about a week, do them 3 times. Also, engage in the aerobic activity that causes you the least strain. That's walking for most pain sufferers, but it can be swimming or any other exercise to increase cardiovascular endurance. Try them out.

*For upper back and neck pain,* emphasize *exercises to increase flexibility 5, 6, and 7* and *exercises to increase strength 5, 6, and 7.* Repeat these exercises twice; then, after about a week, 3 times. After trying out several aerobic exercises, choose those that cause the least strain.

*For the pain of migraine,* emphasize the same exercises as *for upper back and neck pain,* since neck pain frequently plays a part in this form of headache.

*For the pain of arthritis,* emphasize *exercises to increase flexibility* for affected areas. Gentle finger or wrist stretches can be added if those areas are affected. The key to exercising to alleviate the pain of arthritis is the gradual progression of movement.

## EXERCISES YOU CAN DO AWAY FROM HOME

You can adapt some of the basic exercises to a sitting position and do them in your parked car or at your office desk. Should a headache strike, the neck-muscle exercise will be particularly helpful. You will, of course, have practiced your basic exercises in your home.

If you feel that doing your basic exercises at work will make you too conspicuous, consider doing the following three which won't call much attention to yourself. They can be used as fill-ins until you can get back to your regular regimen.

*A breathing relaxation exercise.* Sit in a comfortable upright position. Breathe slowly and deeply from your diaphragm, filling your lungs with tobacco-smoke-free air each time. Repeat 15 times.

*A muscle relaxation exercise.* While sitting, bend your head forward and push your chin against your throat as far as possible. Repeat 10 times.

*A general relaxation exercise.* While sitting, breathe slowly and deeply, and s-t-r-e-t-c-h your arms, hands, and fingers, feet, lower legs, and toes.

The exercises I have suggested are simple, easy to do, and, if performed regularly, can be effective against pain when used in conjunction with the other techniques of your pain-control program. But there is a vast variety of pain-control exercises, and some may be more effective for *you*. It's a good idea to have your supervising physician recommend a physical therapist to set up a personalized program to meet your special needs.

# 5

# Total Relaxation Techniques That Work

---

**PAGE GUIDE TO INSTRUCTIONS
FOR USING TOTAL RELAXATION TECHNIQUES
IN YOUR PAIN-CONTROL PROGRAM**

Can you control any of these functions of your body at will, the way you control your muscles?

Your blood pressure
Your heart beat
Your skin temperature
Your perspiration
Your emotional state

If you said no to any of these, you would be agreeing with the medical wisdom of the fairly recent past that put all those functions beyond your control. They were seen as the work of your involuntary nervous system, which does as it sees fit and is invulnerable to your voluntary decisions.

But a revolution has occurred in medical thinking. Now it is agreed that some major functions of the so-called involuntary nervous system are, indeed, subject to your control. Among those are the five functions just named, functions that play an important part in managing your pain.

Each of those functions can be an indicator of stress—*high* blood pressure, *rapid* heart beat, *low* skin temperature, *excess* perspiration, *disturbed* emotional state. You can compel each indicator back to normal, diminish your stress, and since stress and pain are inseparable partners, diminish your pain. You can control the "uncontrollables" with techniques developed and perfected in pain-control centers worldwide through deep relaxation techniques, which I prefer to call total relaxation techniques because they relax the whole body and the whole brain.

## WHAT TOTAL RELAXATION TECHNIQUES HAVE DONE FOR OTHERS

Meet Don Archer. He's in his early forties, an overworked life insurance salesman, overfamilied, with two children from his second marriage, three from his first, and over his head in debt. Playing touch football with buddies from his company, he slipped, yanked his head backward, and writhed with pain. It didn't stop. It didn't let up. It went on day after day after day. Already overburdened by the stress of everyday life, Don also had to bear the crushing stress of pain.

He went to doctors, many of them, and tried everything they prescribed. But three years after his accident, yoked to a neck brace, dependent on painkilling drugs that grew less and less effective as the dosages grew larger and larger, Don faced a life of worsening, and incurable, chronic pain.

In about 1965, Don was in the office of still another doctor, who told him about a new therapy. In the last few years it had worked for chronic-pain patients of other doctors, and for some of his patients. It sounded like a strange therapy to Archer: no drugs, no surgery, no medical machines. It had something to do with deep breathing and a lot to do with the mind, and if Don hadn't been at the end of his rope, he would have thought it was nonsense and said, "No way." But he agreed to try it as part of a total pain-control program. It was a total relaxation technique.

A year later he wore no neck brace. He was off drugs. Today he plays touch football with his buddies. He has scored over pain.

But sometimes when his day has been too long, when too many prospects have said no, when unpaid bills pile up on his desk, and when five kids make his suburban home seem like the New York subway at rush hour, the pain knifes into his neck again. Then he retires to his room, shuts the door, disconnects the phone, goes through his total relaxation technique, and comes back to his family—and to his world—with his stress relieved, pain-free, and feeling that he can take anything anybody dishes out, smiling.

Don Archer is a composite of many chronic-pain victims helped by total relaxation techniques after they began to achieve medical acceptance in the mid-1960s. Rejected as standard medical procedure before then, they had been a successful component of Eastern medicine for thousands of years.

The breakthrough to American medical-establishment approval came mainly as a result of clinical studies conducted at Harvard Medical School and Beth Israel Hospital, Boston, by Dr. Herbert Benson and associate Keith Wallace. Applying the most popular of Eastern total relaxation techniques, transcendental meditation (TM), these investigators observed sharp declines of a blatant barometer of stress, high blood pressure.

Dr. Benson then, in collaboration with psychologist Dr. Patricia Harrington, set up an experiment to test the effectiveness of TM on the total stress syndrome—the impact of all the indicators of stress combined. Using psychological tests that measure stress, the Benson-Harrington team established that New York Telephone

Company workers who practiced TM were less stressed after several months than workers who did not. Stress was dramatically lowered from "the border of the clinical range"—that is, from the stress levels of psychiatric outpatient—"to the middle of the normal range."

That stress could be controlled by a total relaxation technique was confirmed by other investigators using a different technique. Measuring each of the five major indicators of stress after one total relaxation technique, they verified that blood pressure declined, racing hearts slowed down, chilly hands warmed up, perspiration dried, and the brain's electrical printout switched from beta waves (stress and anxiety) to alpha waves (alert relaxation).

With stress control comes a measure of pain control—in a total pain-control program, often a large measure. A total relaxation technique (three others join TM in this chapter) can help you gain control over both.

## WHAT WE'VE LEARNED ABOUT TOTAL RELAXATION TECHNIQUES AT THE PAIN ALLEVIATION CENTER

Total relaxation techniques are essential to the success of our total pain-control program. While it is not a common outcome, they *have* completely relieved pain during the course of an exercise. These techniques commonly account for 20 to 80 percent of pain relief in all types of chronic pain. In particular, excellent results have been obtained in alleviating the pain of migraine and muscle spasms. In addition, patients report that total relaxation induces a long-lingering state of well-being that provides heightened confidence in the fight against stress and pain—confidence that could help to win a victory over both.

In this chapter I will pass on to you what we've learned about total relaxation techniques in ways that you can use comfortably at home or away. You'll learn about four such techniques and how to experiment with them, while helping decrease stress and pain, until you settle on the one that suits you best. They are deep breathing, conditioned relaxation, transcendental meditation, and biofeedback. First you'll learn how they work, and then the simple exercises that will make them work for you.

## HOW TOTAL RELAXATION
## TECHNIQUES WORK

Basically, all total relaxation techniques work by influencing the so-called involuntary nervous system to switch off the body's state of stress. This seems to occur when just one indicator of stress, say, shallow, rapid breathing, is normalized to slow, deep breathing. Then, it appears, all the indicators of stress return to their nonstress state.

While the mechanism of this healthful transformation is not yet understood, it possibly involves a new balance of neurotransmitters in the brain. Serotonin and gamma-aminobutyric acid (GABA), the antistress neurotransmitters, may obtain dominance over the stress neurotransmitters NE and DA. At the same time, the preponderance of serotonin and GABA may stimulate the production of significant quantities of endorphins.

Brief descriptions of the four major total relation techniques follow. Although all share a fundamental similarity and some overlap, some work better for some people than for others. This introduction will lead to the step-by-step techniques later in the chapter. If you're approaching this therapy with a sense of skepticism—"How in the world can deep breathing help my stress and pain?"—one of these techniques, biofeedback, will show you how to observe the physical changes in some of your body's indicators of stress.

### Deep Breathing

Deep breathing is the simplest and perhaps oldest of the total relaxation techniques. Its effectiveness has passed into folklore wisdom. There's not a language in the world in which the average person's prescription to counter stress doesn't translate to "Calm down—take a deep breath."

*Take* a deep breath. Now. It's easy. Just put down this book. Lean back in your chair. Make yourself comfortable. And breathe in . . . deeply . . . from your diaphragm. Then breathe out . . . slow and easy . . . the way nature intended. How does it feel? Great, right? If it's so good, try it again. Close your eyes this time, and continue to breathe . . . in, out . . . in, out . . . slowly . . . easily . . . in, out . . . in, out . . . Feeling wonderful? Imagine how much better you'll feel when you learn the fine points of deep breathing later in this chapter.

## Conditioned Relaxation

A deep breathing exercise takes about twenty minutes, but you can achieve the same result with just one "command breath" after you've trained yourself in deep breathing.

This technique is based on the classic experiment of the Russian Nobel laureate, Dr. Ivan Pavlov. When he showed meat to dogs, they salivated. He rang a bell at the same time. Meat/bell . . . salivation. After many sessions, he just rang the bell. Bell . . . salivation. The dogs salivated *without* the meat. This psychological device is known as conditioning, and Dr. David E. Bressler was the first to apply it to deep breathing.

At the beginning of each deep-breathing exercise, he taught his patients to take a special kind of breath (that's the "bell") and then to go on to the twenty-minute exercise (that's the "meat"). Special breath/deep-breathing exercise . . . total relaxation. After many sessions, he told his patients just to take the special breath. Special breath . . . total relaxation. His patients went into a state of total relaxation *without* the deep-breathing exercise.

Dr. Bressler, who calls this instant relaxation conditioned relaxation, advises, "if you feel a sudden surge of pain or stress while driving on the freeway, you would be unable to perform an entire [deep-breathing] exercise . . . but it would certainly be possible to take a quick breath that would immediately induce relaxation."

## Transcendental Meditation (TM)

A drawback of deep breathing is that it doesn't always shut out stressful thought patterns while you're performing the exercise. These almost always sabotage the effects of the relaxation technique. TM is usually deep breathing with an additional feature that minimizes or eliminates the sabotaging thoughts.

This is what might happen to you during a deep breathing exercise without TM:

You're leaning back comfortably in your chair, eyes closed, breathing deeply, rhythmically, and naturally from your diaphragm when thoughts intrude and career through your brain. If you're like most of us, the thoughts involve worries, concerns, failures, problems, even pain. They're stress thoughts. They speak to your involuntary system directly, just as your deep breathing is doing, but their voice, compared to that of the deep breathing, is like a thunderclap against a whisper. Stress dominates. Your deep breathing is overwhelmed. You give up.

But TM banishes virtually all stressful thought patterns (indeed, *all* thought patterns, because even the relaxed ones lead to stressful ones) with a simple device. As you expel each deep breath, say to yourself silently the word *one.* Focusing your attention on that word permits no thoughts, or only a few manageable thoughts, to enter your consciousness. Deep breathing can thus work unimpeded.

Make a trial run right now. Start deep breathing. The stressful thoughts rush in. Counter with *one* at every expiration of your breath. Almost at once you can feel the thoughts breaking up, retreating, leaving you. With practice, you can chase stressful thoughts away for the entire exercise.

TM can also be employed without deep breathing. Just go to a quiet place, seat yourself comfortably, close your eyes, and repeat *one* over and over. With stressful thoughts dispelled, your body and brain are likely to settle back into total relaxation that could help to dispel your pain.

## Biofeedback

Deep breathing. Reciting *one* ritualistically. *That's* the way to beat pain? *Chronic* pain? The *worst pain* of all? If you're like most Americans who have been brought up on the scalpel and the pill as modern medicine's only weapons against illness, you'll find it beyond belief. But without belief, you would never be able to stay with the twenty-minute sessions, time and time again, that lead to the end of pain. Biofeedback provides you with that belief.

Biofeedback, explains clinical psychologist Dr. Ken Pelletier, one of the vanguard scientists who introduced the technique in the early 1970s, is TM hooked up to a monitoring device. As one or another of your body's indicators of stress reverses toward normal, the monitoring device flashes or buzzes or swings its meter dial or even plays triumphant music. You have the evidence of your senses, backed by your faith in instrumentation, that TM is producing tangible results, real results—that it is, truly, working for you.

In a typical example, you may not notice the tiny puddles of perspiration with which stress dots your skin. But the monitor to which your skin is wired *does* notice, and it tells you that it does when a light pops on. But when TM does its job, the perspiration dries up, and the light pops off. So does stress.

"But stress is one thing, pain is another," patients say. "Can biofeedback convince me—give me real evidence—that TM cut down my pain?" Quite often. Consider this.

You're suffering from migraine. You're told by your doctor that sudden changes in the pressure of the blood vessels surrounding your brain is the cause of the throbbing pain. As TM takes over, the reading on the thermometric device attached to your hand shows a warming trend. That means that blood which might have put pressure on your brain is flowing into your hand. As you watch the temperature rise, you feel your pain decline.

"What's truly wonderful about feedback," many of our patients tell us, "is that now I know for sure, and you doctors know for sure, that my pain is real, that it isn't 'just in my head.' " A great fear of many patients is that chronic pain is imaginery. But when they actually observe evidence of its existence on a monitor, the fear of mental illness vanishes, and that relieves another major stress, which in turn relieves pain.

Patients also learn something most of them had doubted—that the brain can influence pain. In a state of total relaxation, as they watch a stress-indicator monitor (think of the speedometer of your car), they discover to their amazement that they can alter the readings at will (as you can change the speed of your car). Hand temperatures, for example, go up and down at their command. With practice, they're even able to raise the temperature of one finger while lowering the temperature of the finger next to it.

This control of pain and stress—the control of "involuntary" bodily functions—is the final proof, dramatically convincing, that the total relaxation techniques *do* work. Patients who came to us as disbelievers leave us as fervent apostles.

But you don't have to practice biofeedback on the expensive instruments at pain-control centers, although it's a good idea to start on them. You can start with no equipment at all by monitoring your own pulse. You can use a piece of familiar household equipment, a mirror, to observe the smoothing out of the furrows on your brow. Or you can purchase a low-cost ring thermometer, which we recommend for its easily observed readings, which will feed back impressive evidence of the surges of blood under your command.

Remember, though, that biofeedback is the "convincer" that TM and other total relaxation techniques work, not a technique. It's the proof of the therapy, not the therapy. It's a way to bring you to acceptance of total relaxation techniques as a valid standard medical technique for the alleviation of stress and pain. But once accepted, once at least one of the total relaxation techniques has become part of your pain-control program, you have no further need for biofeedback. You have complete confidence that your mind can help you conquer pain.

"Why use a machine," asks Dr. Herbert Benson, "for something you can do naturally?"

---

## INSTRUCTIONS FOR USING
## TOTAL RELAXATION TECHNIQUES

Try the first three techniques in the order in which they appear. After a few sessions of each, add biofeedback. It will convince you that you're on the right track and speed your learning. When you have experienced the first three techniques, select the one that suits you best. Use biofeedback to supply you with an uplifting dose of assurance whenever you need it.

### Deep Breathing

Exercise time: 20 minutes, twice daily

#### Getting Ready

1. Select the most pleasant room in your home. Advise your family that you are about to practice your total relaxation technique and are not to be disturbed. Be sure the phone is turned off and that no household sounds can come through the closed door. Lighting should be subdued.
2. Wear loose clothing. Remove your wristwatch and jewelry. Remove your eyeglasses or contact lenses. Feel unburdened . . . free.
3. Sit down in a cozy chair and make yourself comfortable. Close your eyes. Become conscious of your breathing.

#### The Deep-Breathing Exercise

1. Breathe through your nose in your natural rhythm, slowly and deeply, drawing in your breath from your diaphragm. You know you're doing it right when your stomach moves up and down.

---

2. Place total concentration on your breathing. Nothing else exists except . . . *in, out* . . . *in, out* . . . *in, out* . . .
3. Continue for 20 minutes.
4. Open your eyes slowly as you return to your regular breathing pattern. You should be deeply refreshed, feeling less stress and less pain.

### What to Watch For

1. If you find stray thoughts wandering into your mind, try to get rid of them with this technique. Imagine a bright star. It's the only star in the heavens. Focus on it with intense concentration. Continue your deep breathing.
2. If you feel you can relax better lying down, don't. Deep breathing is so relaxing that you may fall asleep before you complete the session. (But remember this technique when you can't fall asleep at night.)
3. If you miss your deep breathing session at home, go through it in your parked car or in a quiet place at work, if you can find one.

## Conditioned Relaxation

Exercise time: 20 minutes, twice daily.

### Getting Ready

1. Repeat steps 1 through 3 of Deep Breathing, Getting Ready (page 62).

### The Conditioned Relaxation Exercise

1. The "command breath." Breathe out through your mouth. Take a deep breath through your mouth. Breathe out through your nose.

   Later on this breath will command your body and brain to go into total relaxation. Do not repeat this command breath until step 3.

2. Repeat steps 1 through 4 of Deep Breathing, the deep-breathing exercise (page 62).
3. After two weeks of successful deep-breathing exercises, just take the command breath—that's all. You should be conditioned to go into total relaxation.

### What to Watch For

1. Everything listed under this heading for Deep Breathing (page 63).

## Transcendental Meditation (TM)

Exercise time: 20 minutes, twice daily.

### Getting Ready

1. Repeat steps 1 through 3 of Deep Breathing, Getting Ready (page 62).

### The Transcendental Meditation Exercise

1. Breathe through your nose according to your natural rhythm, slowly and deeply, drawing in your breath from your diaphragm as you did in your deep-breathing exercise, but with this difference: As you breathe out, recite the word *one* silently, stretching out the syllable—*woooonnnnn*—to last as long as the exhalation.
2. Place total concentration on the drawn-out syllable. Nothing exists except *woooonnnnn . . . woooonnnnn . . . woooonnnnn . . .* Continue for 20 minutes.
3. Open your eyes slowly as you discontinue reciting *woooonnnnn* and return to your regular breathing pattern. As with deep breathing alone, you should be deeply refreshed and feel less stress and less pain.

## *What to Watch For*

1. If you're uncomfortable reciting the word *one,* substitute any word that suits you. Actually, the word *one* is an Americanization of *oom,* the word most frequently employed by Hindu TM adepts.
2. If thoughts continue to stray through your brain, do not make a *conscious* effort to shut them out. The more you try, the tighter they'll stick. They'll also spread out into a tangled spiderweb of stressful thoughts that could strangle the exercise. Just ignore your stray thoughts, continue to focus attention on the word of your choice (your mantra), and they'll fade away before they can do any damage.
3. If you can't handle both deep breathing and your mantra simultaneously, try only the mantra after Getting Ready. Just by shutting out your stressful thoughts, you can reduce your stress and consequently your pain. Some patients report that when they practice only the mantra, deep breathing occurs spontaneously after several sessions.

## Biofeedback

Exercise time: about 25 minutes

### *Getting Ready*

1. For this exercise, place a thermometer ring on your ring finger. It is an inexpensive item that can be obtained at most pharmacies.
2. Jot down your finger temperature.

### *The Biofeedback Technique Exercise*

1. Practice any of the total relaxation techniques described in this chapter.
2. When you are through, take a reading of the ring thermometer. The temperature will have gone up.

3. Daydream about a warmer finger (for instance, see in your mind your finger dangling in a basin of warm water) and watch the thermometer rise.

   You will have reversed an indicator of stress, hand coldness. If you suffer from migraine, as the temperature of your finger increases, your pain will decrease.

4. After several sessions, try to raise your finger temperature only by daydreaming. Your daydream acts like a mantra, and the ring thermometer will indicate a rise in temperature.

### *What to Watch For*

1. If you can't obtain a ring thermometer, take your pulse before and after the exercise. Not only will it slow down, it will slow down even more as you daydream about its happening. Or simply observe the worry lines on your forehead in a mirror before and after the exercise.

2. If you have trouble daydreaming, start by putting your thoughts in the form of a wish—"I wish my hands were in thick warm gloves" or "I wish I were warming my hands over a blazing log fire," and so on—then visualize its happening.

# 6

# Mind Over Pain:
# Two Proven Techniques

Long before neurobiologists understood that certain biochemicals in the brain, the endorphins fight pain, two techniques of mind control were stimulating the production of those substances. Now part of standard pain-control programs, the techniques are autogenics and self-hypnosis.

## Autogenics

This word translates roughly into "produced by oneself" or "produced from within" as opposed to produced by outside influences such as doctors and drugs. It originated as part of a medical movement that placed heavy emphasis on the body's capacity to heal itself. Created in Germany by Dr. Wolfgang Luthe and Dr. Johannes Schultz in the late 1920s, autogenics was the subject of more than two thousand studies in that country before it began to be adopted by American pain specialists about a decade ago.

Autogenics is a technique for freeing the mind from conscious thought so it can operate freely on its unconscious level. It is on that level, Luthe and Schultz held, that the brain naturally directs repairs of damage to a human being, restoring the body to a normal, healthy, pain-free state.

The autogenic technique is essentially a mixture of three total relaxation techniques. It is a variation of transcendental meditation, to shut off conscious thought. It is also a method of reversing some indicators of stress, to induce the state of total relaxation in which the unconscious mind works at its best. It is, finally, a form of biofeedback, with parts of the human body acting as feedback machines. Its overriding plus is that it is extremely simple to use.

## Self-Hypnosis

Like autogenics, self-hypnosis is a technique for switching off the conscious mind and switching on the unconscious mind. It differs from autogenics in that it does not leave the unconscious mind to carry out its healing function unassisted. Self-hypnosis provides stimulation and even guidance.

While the healing power of hypnosis has been recognized for ages in almost all cultures, it wasn't until 1958 that the American Medical Association approved courses in that discipline in medical schools. Since then, however, hypnosis has been accepted as an adjunct therapy in the management of some maladies, of which chronic pain is the most prominent.

Hypnosis, despite its widespread association in the public mind with a professional hypnotist who is an entertainer, is basically a do-it-yourself technique. Only you can activate the bioneurological mechanism that closes the door of the conscious and opens the door to the unconscious workings of the brain. The hypnotist—today called the hypnotherapist—simply prompts you to push-button the mechanism. But you don't need prompting from anyone else; you can be your own prompter. Entering the hypnotic state by yourself has the advantages of relieving you of dependence on the hypnotherapist, saving you fees, giving you the lift that comes with a sense of personal achievement, and reinforcing the feeling that what you do for yourself is more effective than what a hypnotherapist can do for you.

Self-hypnosis is a superalert state of the unconscious mind. There's no theatrical trance, no more loss of touch with the world around you than you experience at an absorbing movie. Your conscious brain is, after a fashion, slumbering, but your unconscious brain is wide awake, keenly attentive to the needs of your body for the restoration and maintenance of its good health.

Your unconscious mind is wide open, ultrasensitive to your demands for improved health, and rapidly responsive to them. When you call for a stop to pain, the endorphins—which cannot be controlled by your conscious mind—start to flow. They bring relief from pain, relief that can last long after the self-hypnotic session is over.

## WHAT MIND-OVER-PAIN TECHNIQUES HAVE DONE FOR OTHERS

A voluminous body of scientific literature attests to the efficacy of autogenics as a total relaxation technique that relieves stress, and consequently pain, directly by the promotion of endorphins in the brain. Observers report that autogenics is particularly helpful in alleviating the pain of migraine.

Self-hypnosis lends itself to more varied strategies in the fight against pain, based on the unconscious mind's ultrasensitivity under hypnosis to your needs for better health. The expression of those needs is called, in psychological parlance, hypnotic suggestion. Here's a sampling of those suggestions that, weird as they may seem, work.

Sara's hypnotic suggestion was for the fierce pain in her head to go to her knuckles instead. It did. There was no difference in the intensity of the pain, but it was easier for her to bear it in her knuckles than in her head.

Norman's hypnotic suggestion was for the long, virtually sleepless nights while he suffered agonizing back pain to pass rapidly. They did—or seemed to. To Norman, the long nights whisked by in minutes.

Earl's hypnotic suggestion was for the feelings of fear and anxiety that made his postoperative pain worse to be replaced by feelings of security and calm. They were, and his pain declined.

Tricia's hypnotic suggestion was for the sharp, cutting pain that was disrupting her life to be replaced by a pleasant feeling, as if she were being massaged. It was.

Can hypnotic suggestion quite directly stop pain? Many reliable reports state that for some individuals it can. One pain-control authority has characterized hypnotic suggestion as the most potent way of ending chronic pain.

## WHAT WE'VE LEARNED ABOUT MIND-OVER-PAIN TECHNIQUES AT THE PAIN ALLEVIATION CENTER

We have found both autogenics and self-hypnosis to be effective pain-control techniques when employed as elements of a total pain-control program.

Autogenics, which is comparatively easy to learn and perform, is most effective in cases of moderate pain. Self-hypnosis, which requires patience to master, has produced excellent results in severe cases of chronic pain. Our patients most often obtain pain relief by making the hypnotic suggestion that their pain, no matter how torturous, is just a tingling sensation, and that's all they feel.

In this chapter you'll find explanations of how both mind-over-pain techniques work, followed by step-by-step instructions for making them work for you. Including both techniques in your pain-control program is a more potent method than trying either one alone. But if one doesn't suit you, be sure to give the other a chance.

## HOW MIND-OVER-PAIN
## TECHNIQUES WORK

*The autogenic technique* consists of the repetition of each of six formulas:

1. My arms and legs are heavy.
2. My arms and legs are warm.
3. My heartbeat is calm and regular.
4. My breathing is calm and regular.
5. My abdomen is warm.
6. My forehead is cool.

The formulas, when they are recited over and over again, act as mantras, shutting out thoughts, particularly stressful thoughts, that interfere with your communications to the unconscious level of the brain. It is on this level that the so-called involuntary actions, including those associated with stress and pain, take place. Getting your messages through to that level can help control just the involuntary actions that are related to the reduction of both stress and pain.

In autogenics, the basic involuntary actions subject to your control are blood flow and respiration. Reciting, "My arms and legs . . . my abdomen . . . are warm . . . heavy," causes blood to gush to them. Reciting, "My forehead is cool," causes blood to rush away. Reciting "My heartbeat is calm and regular," causes the rate of blood flow to be carefully regulated. Your respiration obeys your command as you recite, "My breathing is calm and regular."

Autogenics works to reverse two prime indicators of stress. The chaotic irregularity of the bloodstream under stress is soothed into placid normality. The stress-induced short, hectic gasps for air are tranquilized into smooth and serene breathing. The transposition of these two indicators of stress reverses—as you should already know—the total stress syndrome, bringing about a state of total relaxation, which lowers stress and pain.

It is probably good that the repetition of each of the six formulas induces a hypnotic state, and the directives of the formulas have all the force of hypnotic suggestion. It is an easily monitored force, for the biofeedback of the body is rapid and obvious. You *feel* that your arms and legs are heavy. You *feel* that your arms and legs are warm. You *feel* that your heartbeat is calm and regular. You *feel* that your abdomen is warm. You *feel* that your forehead is cool. From what you *feel,* you know that autogenics is working.

There are physiological reasons, too, that may explain the success of autogenics. Its capability of moving blood from the head, as evidenced by a temperature drop ("My forehead is cool"), is a tactic for combating migraine, which is caused by changes in pressure in the vessels surrounding the brain. Its capability of oxygenating blood optimally ("My breathing is calm and regular) and carrying that excess blood to pain-prone regions of the body, as evidenced by a temperature rise ("My arms and legs are warm" . . . "My abdomen is warm"), may help fight pain with an abundance of blood substances and oxygen.

Pain relief from autogenics may come as well, according to the speculations of its creators, by permitting the unconscious part of the brain to proceed with its work of restoring health without the impediment of conscious thought. The unconscious mind, then, directs the release of endorphins to restore a pain-free body.

*The self-hypnotic technique* involves total muscular relaxation through mental control. At first you focus your mind on relaxing all your muscles simultaneously, then, in turn, the muscles of your feet, calves, thighs, stomach, chest, back, neck, shoulders, and arms. Accompanied by deep breathing, this creates a state of total relaxation, which in itself helps ease your stress and pain.

At the same time, this technique presses the OFF button on your conscious brain and the ON button on your unconscious brain. (The nature of these "buttons" is yet to be discovered, but an educated guess, based on recent research with hypnotic drugs, would involve some neurotransmitters, the substances that make the brain work.) When your unconscious is on, it is wide open to your suggestions—suggestions to which your unconscious mind would never listen, let alone heed, if you were not in the hypnotic state. You can make two general types of effective suggestions concerning your pain.

The first is "Get rid of my pain." Your unconscious mind will attempt to do this by boosting the flow of endorphins during hypnosis; this is called hypnotic suggestion.

The second type of suggestion is "From now on, when I'm not in hypnosis, get rid of my pain whenever I count from one to ten." This is called posthypnotic suggestion. It occurs *after* the hypnosis.

That one-to-ten count is a sort of code that triggers your unconscious brain (think of it in this instance as a computer) to replay the directions for increased endorphin flow that had been given under hypnosis. Your unconscious mind had stored the code in its memory bank and left a channel of communication open to receive it.

Counting to ten may be one way you can rely on to relieve your pain.

---

### INSTRUCTIONS FOR USING
### MIND-OVER-PAIN TECHNIQUES
**Because autogenics is an excellent preparation for self-hypnosis, practice it first.**

#### Autogenics

Exercise time: about 5 minutes, twice daily

*Getting Ready*

1. During the exercise, you will recite the six autogenic formulas (page 71) to yourself silently, slowly, and rhythmically, like an incantation. You can tape-record them before the ex-

ercise, then play them back during the exercise for guidance. Or—the better way—you can memorize them.
2. Repeat all steps under Deep Breathing, Getting Ready (page 62)
3. Breathe deeply (page 62) about 6 times, then begin the exercise. Continue to breathe deeply during the exercise.

### The Autogenic Exercise

1. Recite each of the following formulas silently 6 times. If you're using a tape as guide, synchronize your recitations with your voice on the tape. Before you begin a new formula, count slowly from 1 to 10.

> *"My arms and legs are heavy."*
> *"My arms and legs are warm."*
> *"My heartbeat is calm and regular."*
> *"My breathing is calm and regular."*
> *"My abdomen is warm."*
> *"My forehead is cool."*

2. Rest quietly for a minute or so while you enjoy the total relaxation experience and savor the joy of lessened pain. Open your eyes slowly, rise gently, and reenter the conscious world with a new sense of well-being.

### What to Watch For

1. If the physiological effects are too intense—you may feel too heavy or too warm or too cool—change the formula to describe effects that are right for you. For example, instead of saying "heavy," say "heavy, but not too heavy."
2. If your muscles twitch during your first autogenic exercises, don't worry. This is a harmless reaction that will undoubtedly disappear as you become accustomed to the technique.
3. If you feel faint, dizzy, or disoriented at the end of the exercise, it may be that your reentry into the conscious world is too abrupt. Be sure to follow step 2 of The Autogenic Exercise.

## Self-Hypnosis

Exercise time: 20 minutes daily

***Caution:*** You may not be hypnotizable. The doctor supervising your program may want to recommend a hypnotherapist who will determine if you are (most people are). Your initial experience with hypnosis should be with a hypnotherapist who can ease you over the rough spots and make you feel at home with the technique.

### *Getting Ready*

1. In the following exercise, you will be your own hypnotherapist, using phrases similar to those your hypnotherapist used. You can memorize those phrases and recite them to yourself silently, or you can record them and play them back. Since the tone of your voice—it should be soothing and compelling—is a factor in the effectiveness of the hypnotic technique, you might try several rehearsals, speaking aloud without recording items 1 through 12 of The Self-Hypnosis Technique, which follows. Then record.
2. Repeat all the steps of Deep Breathing, Getting Ready (page 62).
3. Breathe deeply (page 62) about 6 times, then begin the self-hypnosis technique, preferably breathing deeply throughout the exercise.

### *The Self-hypnosis Technique*

Repeat the following instructions to yourself silently, or listen to them on the tape you've prepared.

1. You're relaxing. You're squeezing the stiffness out of your muscles. Feel them soften. They're becoming slack. They're like unstretched rubber bands. They're loose. They're hanging. They're limp. Your whole body is loose . . . it's hanging . . . it's limp. You're feeling relaxed . . . more and more relaxed . . . so pleasantly relaxed.

2. Think of your feet. See them in your mind's eye. They're still a little stiff. Let the muscles of your feet go limp . . . totally limp. Let them get heavier . . . and heavier . . . and, oh, so much heavier. How relaxed your feet feel!

3. Think of your whole body. See it in your mind's eye. It's more relaxed . . . more and more relaxed.

4. Think of your calves and thighs. See them in your mind's eye. They're still a little stiff. Let the muscles of your calves and thighs go limp . . . totally limp. Let them get heavier . . . and heavier . . . and, oh, so much heavier. How relaxed your calves and thighs feel!

5. Think of your whole body. See it in your mind's eye. It's more relaxed . . . more and more relaxed.

6. Think of your stomach muscles. See them in your mind's eye. They're still a little stiff. Let your stomach muscles go limp . . . totally limp. Let them get heavier . . . and heavier . . . and, oh, so much heavier. How relaxed your stomach muscles feel!

7. Think of your whole body. See it in your mind's eye. It's more relaxed . . . more and more relaxed.

8. Think of your chest muscles and your back muscles. They're still a little stiff. Let your chest muscles and your back muscles go limp . . . totally limp. Let them get heavier . . . and heavier . . . and, oh, so much heavier. How relaxed your chest muscles and your back muscles feel!

9. Think of your whole body. See it in your mind's eye. It's more relaxed . . . more and more relaxed.

10. Think of your arms muscles. They're still a little stiff. Let your arm muscles go limp . . . totally limp. Let them get heavier . . . and heavier and, oh, so much heavier. How relaxed your arm muscles feel!

11. Think of your whole body. See it in your mind's eye. It's more relaxed . . . more and more relaxed. Think of your feet. See them in your mind's eye. How relaxed they are! Think of your calves and thighs. See them in your mind's eye. How relaxed they are! Think of your stomach muscles. See them in your mind's eye. How relaxed they are! Think of your chest muscles and your back muscles. See them in your

mind's eye. How relaxed they are. Think of your arm muscles. See them in your mind's eye. How relaxed they are. See
your whole body in your mind's eye. It's so relaxed . . . sooo
relaxed . . . You've never felt it soooooooo relaxed.

*(Do not recite this section. It is included here to tell you what's
happening. At this point of the exercise, you are in the hypnotic
state, with a direct line open to your unconscious mind, which is
intensely susceptible to suggestion. You will now suggest that
your pain be transformed to just a tingle, and then you will plant
the posthypnotic suggestion that it will become a tingle again
whenever you count from 1 to 10 anywhere, anyplace, without
going into the hypnotic state. Continue to talk to yourself—on
tape or silently. And remember, the "you" you're talking to is
your unconscious mind.)*

12. Your pain is growing weaker . . . weaker and weaker . . . It's
    just a pleasant tingle.
13. From now on your pain will become a pleasant tingle when-
    ever you count 1 . . . 2 . . . 3 . . . 4 . . . 5 . . . 6 . . . 7 . . . 8 . . .
    9 . . . 10.
14. When you count backwards from 3 to 1, you will wake up
    refreshed and feeling great. 3 . . . 2 . . . 1. Open your eyes
    gradually. Get up slowly. Flex your muscles.
15. When the hypnotic effect wears off and you feel pain again,
    test your posthypnotic suggestion. Count 1 . . . 2 . . . 3 . . . 4
    . . . 5 . . . 6 . . . 7 . . . 8 . . . 9 . . . 10.

### What to Watch For

1. If your attempts at self-hypnosis are unsuccessful at first,
   don't give up. It takes patience and motivation to master this
   technique. Think positively, stick to it, and keep your goal in
   mind: to downgrade your pain to a pleasant tingle and up-
   grade your life.
2. If you're tempted to give up the rest of your pain-control program for a quick fix of self-hypnotism, *don't*. Self-hypnosis
   stimulates endorphin flow, which reduces your pain, but it

does not necessarily remove other causes of your pain. Your pain control program is aimed at doing that. Besides, self-hypnosis works better within the context of your total program than by itself.

3. If you're concerned about not being able to cope with emergencies while you're under self-hypnosis, reassure yourself by adding this posthypnotic suggestion: "You will wake up fully alert in any emergency situation." In reality, despite the use of traditional commands to "wake up," hypnosis is not sleep, but rather a raised state of unconscious awareness of the body's health needs, which makes it particularly responsive to emergency situations. (The hypnotic command to "wake up" really means to shift your communication with your brain from its unconscious to its conscious region.)

4. If self-hypnosis stirs up forgotten disagreeable memories and feelings—and it may do that—do not proceed without consulting your supervising doctor. You may need psychotherapeutic guidance.

5. If you get the urge to try posthypnotic suggestions in addition to pain control, *don't*. That could lead to disturbed mental states and even increase your pain.

6. If nothing happens when you count from 1 to 10, repeat the exercise.

7. If you are disturbed by the drawbacks of self-hypnosis, don't let that deter you from trying it. Properly monitored by your doctor or by a hypnotherapist or psychotherapist, self-hypnosis is usually a safe and particularly effective pain-control therapy.

# 7

# Pain-Control Imagery: The Movies of the Mind

---

**PAGE GUIDE TO INSTRUCTIONS
FOR USING THE MOVIES OF THE MIND
IN YOUR PAIN-CONTROL PROGRAM**

Can you tell your pain to stop?

Yes, you can, but not with words.

You can do it with images. Images you create in your mind; images that you can guide and direct.

These are the movies of the mind, a recently discovered nonverbal language that your body's pain mechanisms can understand.

# WHAT THE MOVIES OF THE MIND HAVE DONE FOR OTHERS

Margaret Miller was the subject of a crucial pioneering study of the movies of the mind. Around 1975, when she arrived, she came in desperation, at Dr. Martin Rossman's San Francisco clinic, she had suffered the agonies of a tightened urethra since age eleven. The urethra is a tube that carries off urine from the bladder. When it is tightened, the pain of the pressure of the liquid against the wall of the tube is excruciating.

At that time, Dr. Rossman, shocked by the general failure of medical treatment for chronic pain, was attempting to confirm the value of a new, outrageously different therapy. He had suspended his thriving private practice to study under that therapy's creator, Dr. Irving Oyle, at his Bolinias, California, Headlands Healing Service. He had returned to San Francisco enthusiastic about Dr. Oyle's successful results and determined to check it out against the most difficult of his patients.

Dr. Oyle's startling therapy was pain-control imagery. Dr. Rossman's most difficult patient was the newcomer Margaret Miller.

During forty-four years of standard urological treatment, Margaret had never been without pain for a moment, and the pain had grown more and more horrible. Pronounced by the latest of a long line of urologists as incurable—"You'll just have to learn to live with your pain"—Margaret was the ideal subject for Dr. Rossman's study. If *she* could be relieved of her pain, Dr. Rossman thought, then Dr. Oyle's therapy would be indisputably proved.

Dr. Rossman trained Margaret Miller to project her own movie of the mind. Relaxed, with her eyes closed, she pictured her bladder and drops of water falling into it. The drops fell gently, ever so gently, and her bladder puffed up slowly, like a toy balloon. When her bladder was full, Margaret saw a stream of liquid,—very powerful because her bladder was full—flow into her urethra and spread the constricted walls of the tube farther and farther and farther apart until a wide channel had been formed through which the liquid flowed easily, smoothly—and painlessly.

In real life, her urine flowed through her urethra easily, smoothly—and painlessly.

Three years later, Margaret wrote to her urologist. She told him about her movie of the mind—how it had ended her pain, how she continued to view it twice a day, and how the pain had never come back. "He wrote back to me," Margaret said, "that he didn't believe me."

Around 1978, few doctors would have believed her. Even Dr. David E. Bressler, the director of the UCLA Pain Control Unit, who was to become a strong advocate of pain-control imagery, confesses that "when I was . . . introduced to the . . . technique of Dr. Irving Oyle, I was as quick to challenge it as anyone. How could it do all the things he claimed? . . . It was so unorthodox, I doubted if the typical patient would accept it.

Putting it to the test with his own patients, Dr. Bressler was "surprised not only by the immense value of guided imagery [another name for pain-control imagery] but at how receptive most pain sufferers are to the technique . . . [It] has helped them to accomplish what many doctors thought was impossible—a life free of agonizing pain."

Dr. Bressler's conclusion has been strongly affirmed by other clinical investigators, including the following eminent pain-control specialists:

Dr. C. Norman Shealy, founder of the Pain and Rehabilitation Center, La Crosse, Wisconsin, regards movies of the mind as "the number one plan to stop pain. It is the single most effective technique—bar none . . . It works on headaches, backaches, arthritis, and any other kind of pain."

Dr. Neil H. Olshan, director of the Chronic Pain-Control Unit, Mesa Lutheran Hospital, Mesa, Arizona, reports that "83 percent of patients who were taught pain-control imagery reduced their pain by 55 to 100 percent. This is the key," he claims, "to unlocking your pain."

Dr. O. Carl Simonton and his wife, Stephanie Matthews-Simonton, at their Cancer Counseling Center, Fort Worth, Texas, have employed movies of the mind to lessen pain while significantly extending the lives of their patients.

"People who use movies of the mind," sums up Adelaide Bry, a leading psychological authority on guided imagery, "find themselves refusing painkillers."

# WHAT WE'VE LEARNED ABOUT THE MOVIES OF THE MIND AT THE PAIN ALLEVIATION CENTER

We have found this therapy significantly effective as an integral part of our total pain-control program. Typically, we achieve pain relief ranging from 20 to 30 percent to 70 to 80 percent. Some patients obtain 100 percent relief. These figures apply to all types of chronic pain. In one dramatic case, the movies of the mind succeeded when no other treatment could help.

When Ernest Fuller was referred to us by his neurosurgeon, he was seventy-eight years old. A victim of a disease that most doctors thought only surgery could cure, Mr. Fuller was considered too old and in too deteriorated a state of health to enter the operating theater.

The bony sheath around the canal housing his spinal cord had shrunk, pressing in on his nerves and causing unrelenting, agonizing pain. Narcotic analgesics, the prescribed alternate to surgery, which would have opened the bony sheath and relieved the pressure and pain, provided only partial relief over short periods, and their effectiveness was progressively lessening.

We designed Mr. Fuller a program built around movies of the mind. We started with total relaxation techniques, highlighted by biofeedback to dispel his disbelief in the power of the brain over pain. Because we knew that the impact of movies of the mind is blunted by narcotic analgesics, we placed him on our regimen for gradually discontinuing those drugs. As Mr. Fuller began to project his movies of the mind, he underwent physical therapy, which re-strengthened muscles that had virtually wasted away.

At the end of seven months, this comprehensive pain-control program, with movies of the mind at its center, had produced life-altering results. Mr. Fuller's muscles had grown so strong that he was able to discard his walker, walk briskly, and even swim regularly. His vigor was remarkable for a man his age, especially one who had been chronically ill for so long. His overall health was that of a younger man. Best of all, Mr. Fuller reported no pain.

On the basis of our successful experience at the Pain Alleviation Center, and of similar good reports of pain-control specialists worldwide, movies of the mind are included in your pain-control program. In this chapter, you'll find how they work to influence the pain-control mechanism in your body. The simple explanation will bolster your confidence in the technique. Then you'll be given easy-to-follow instructions on how to create and view *your own* movies of the mind to help relieve *your* pain.

## HOW THE MOVIES
## OF THE MIND WORK

*Background.* It's traditional for doctors to regard the brain and the complex network of nerves spreading out from it—the nervous system—as composed of two parts. One part, the voluntary system, is under your control. (When you wish to put this book down, you command your nervous system to instruct your muscles to do so.) The other part, the involuntary system, controls you. (If you're excited by the message of hope in this book, your heart beats a bit faster and your blood pressure rises.)

You can easily communicate with your voluntary nervous system: thoughts become deeds, words become actions. But can you communicate with your involuntary nervous system—tell your heartbeat, your blood pressure, your digestion, your skin temperature, and all the millions of biochemical reactions that go on in your body every second what to do? Up to recently, doctors thought you could not.

But thanks to the discoveries of neurobiologists, scientists who study the nervous system, doctors now know that you can communicate with the so-called involuntary nervous system. Taking their clue from Eastern medicine, which routinely channels the power of the brain to control what were once thought in the West to be uncontrollable actions of the body, the neurobiologists searched for the special language with which the brain talks to the involuntary nervous system—and found it.

It's a language of images—not of thoughts, not of words (which are the expression of thoughts), but moving pictures that you project on an imaginery screen in your brain. They are images that you create and direct—"guided images": the movies of the mind.

With this newly discovered language—actually a universal language that's as old as mankind—you can tell your involuntary nervous system what to do. Of most importance for you, you can order one component of that system—the mechanism that produces the endorphins—to work at maximum capacity. In that way, you can tell your pain to stop. But with *images*. As these patients did.

## Movies of the Mind That Work

Dennis saw his pain as a giant iceberg on his shoulders that melted under a Miami sun. His pain melted, too.

Irma saw her angina as an elephant, sitting on her chest, who grew thinner and thinner as she put him on a diet. Her pain grew easier and easier to bear.

Jeanne saw her pain as a huge logjam pressing against her leg. She saw a river in flood breaking up the jam, carrying the logs away. As it did her pain.

Alfred saw his migraine as a raging forest fire drowned by a torrential rain. As the fire went out, so did his pain.

Susan, after surgery, saw her pain as a vicious dog gnawing at her spine. When she waved a steak, the dog let go of her spine, and her pain let go.

Ronald saw his brain as a red-hot oven. He saw his head encased in ice. As the ice cooled off his brain, the hot pain of his headache cooled down.

Simone saw her pain as a hot, sharp knife plunged into her spine. She saw the knife turn cool, turn into rubber, turn into nothing, and her pain was turned off.

Some movies of the mind are conceived in greater detail. Here, in a typical one, the patient controls her pain by directly stimulating the production of endorphins.

*I see the endorphins pouring out in greater and greater quantities from my brain. They form a river of soothing ointment. As it flows down my neck, and down my back, and into my thighs, I begin to feel better and better. I see hot acid scorching my leg,*

*but when the soothing ointment reaches it, the acid is neutralized
and turns into harmless water. It's cool and comforting water,
water that massages my leg like a Jacuzzi. Wonderful!*

Today, movies of the mind play major roles in soundly re-
searched and tested medical programs that teach pain-stricken
men, women, and even children to communicate with that part of
the involuntary nervous system which controls pain—the endorphin mechanism. Long strings of successes have been recorded at
UCLA's Pain Control Unit; at the Psychosomatic Medicine Clinic in
Berkeley, California; at the Cancer Counseling and Research Center at Fort Worth, Texas; at the Boston Pain Unit; at the Seattle
Pain Unit; at the University of Miami, Florida, Pain Center; at our
own Pain Alleviation Center; and elsewhere throughout the nation.

"However bizarre it might seem," writes Adelaide Bry, "this is
the wave of the future. The new medicine begins where the old
medicine left off—with the patient's own power to heal himself [or
herself]."

## INSTRUCTIONS FOR USING
## THE MOVIES OF THE MIND

The following instructions will teach you how to open communications with your pain, how to project images in your mind,
and finally, how to create your own movies of the mind.

### Opening a Channel of Communication
### to Your Pain

Perform a total relaxation technique before each of the following
training sessions. After you've mastered the techniques of projecting movies in your mind, the preliminary total relaxation
technique will usually not be necessary. The movie of the mind
itself will act as a total relaxation technique.

But for starters, the relaxation technique opens up a direct
line of communication to the involuntary nervous system, en-

abling you to communicate with your endorphin-producing mechanism. The language understood by that mechanism, as well as all other parts of your involuntary nervous system, is guided imagery, the movies of the mind.

## Learning to Project Images in Your Mind

*Time required*: The following sessions should take just a few seconds each. In a total of about 15 minutes spread over several days, you should be able to project images in your mind at will.

*Session 1.* Keep your eyes closed and visualize the cover of this book. At first it will probably appear as a rough sketch. Then let it develop spontaneously. *Do not* think about it. *Do not* try to describe it in words. *Do not* strive for photographic accuracy. As long as you can see the book cover as you remember it, that's fine.

Repeat this exercise 5 times a day until you can summon up the image at will. That should take about 12 sessions.

*Session 2.* Repeat Session 1 with any other object of your choice, say, a bottle. When, after a few sessions, you can project it instantaneously, repeat it with another object, say, an apple. When you're projecting *that* object successfully, try still another, say, a chair . . . and so on.

Project images 5 times a day until you get the hang of it—about 12 sessions.

*Session 3.* Visualize an empty room, then furnish it item by item. Now blank out your image. Wait. Then project the furnished room again, this time completely furnished. You should be able to do this easily in a few seconds the first time you try it.

You have now mastered the technique of imaging stationary things. You've created "still pictures" of the mind. Now go on to create "*moving* pictures."

Visualize objects in motion. Try it with a car. then a train. Then a horse. Then a person. Then many persons. You should have no trouble doing this. In the few seconds it takes, you'll have a lot of fun, plus a sense of achievement. That builds a feel-good state, conducive to fighting pain.

You're now ready to project the movies of your mind.

## Creating Your Own Movies of the Mind

*Time required*: It should take you about 10 minutes to create a feature movie of your mind, but it will take only a few seconds to run it off thereafter. To create a short movie of the mind should take, at most, 5 minutes, and about a second to run it off thereafter.

*Session 4.* Remember that wonderful feeling you had as a child when your mom and dad said they were taking you to the movies? Let the memory unreel in your mind, bringing back that exciting mood of joyous anticipation. Now, feeling "up" and receptive (in itself an enemy of pain), *go* to the movies—the movies of your mind that *you* are going to make from now on.

At this session, make the happy discovery that you have always known how to make movies of your mind, and that you have been doing it right along—*when you daydream.* Think about it. Isn't that so? What you're going to learn is simply *daydreaming with a purpose*—guided daydreaming with guided images to lessen your pain.

Today, you'll daydream about What it will be like when your pain is gone. Here's how a thirty-year-old chronic-back-pain victim with a three-year-old daughter daydreamed it into a feature movie of the mind.

*I see myself playing roughhouse games with my daughter—she loves them—picking her up, tossing her around, rolling over and over with her. I see myself even picking up after her—happily. I see us walking together, running together, swimming together, playing ball together. I see myself going to the supermarket, bending down to pick up gallon bottles from the bottom shelf, reaching up to pluck heavy cans from the top shelf. I see myself jogging, playing tennis, dancing—doing all the things I used to do. I look at myself in close-up. I look different. I look happy.*

Now daydream what it will be like when *your* pain is gone. Remember—no words, images only.

*Session 5.* Create a short movie of your mind, similar to those listed on page 84. They're very useful in situations when you need extra-quick pain relief. Just close your eyes, project your daydream, like the following example, open your eyes in a second or so, and feel the difference.

*I see my pain as a rusty electric saw cutting the bone in my arm. I reach out and press the* STOP *button. The saw stops, and so does my pain.*

### Using Your Own Movies
### of the Mind to Fight Pain

Project your feature movie of the mind twice a day and your short movie of the mind 5 times a day or as often as you need them. After a few weeks you may find that your short movie of the mind alone is sufficient to satisfy your pain-control needs. Deep breathing during the viewing of your movie will improve its effectiveness.

If you have trouble creating your own movie of the mind, try one of the following two methods that have helped others.

### *Prepare a Story Board*

This is a technique that creators of TV commercials use before they put their production before cameras. Think of a story, then draw a series of pictures illustrating it, each showing a change of action. Then run through the sequence rapidly in your mind. The stills turn into motion, and you have made a movie of the mind.

### *Let Your Brain Take Over*

Adelaide Bry describes what happens from her own experience, which, she says, "might be your own as well." When you close your eyes . . .

> *The lights fade. You have a sense of darkness, perhaps empti-*
> *ness. Gradually you notice something. A form. Some movements.*
> *Your movie camera [of your mind] turns toward it. It's not quite*
> *clear yet but you sense what it is. You focus on it. The scene*
> *becomes brighter. Ah, there it is. Not at all what you expected.*
> *Interesting, but not especially meaningful. You're tempted to*
> *open your eyes and forget the whole thing.*
>
> *But you're curious. You decide to go with it. Things begin to*
> *happen. It's fascinating. Also, a little scary. You don't realize*
> *where it's all going to go. You suddenly realize it's your movie*
> *and you can do anything you want with it. You decide to really*
> *let go . . . You can put yourself in the movie, take yourself out,*
> *rewrite the script, and create entirely new situations.*

What images, what situations are right for the relief of your pain?

"You will get to know very clearly when it comes," Bry advises. "It will feel utterly right. You will have no doubt about it at that moment, so you will have a sense of resolution and deep satisfaction."

That deep satisfaction may come only after several tries. It may come at the first try.

As you view *your* movies of the mind, no matter how bizarre they are, you'll feel your pain subsiding. "In the realm of the mind," observes psychotherapist Dr. John Lilly, "what you believe to be true is true.

# 8

# Nutrients That Fight Pain and Depression

Evidence published in 1978 by Dr. Seymour Ehrenpreis, head of a Chicago Medical School research team, that a natural substance in food, a nutrient, could reduce pain opened a new direction in modern medicine's exploration of ways to combat chronic pain.

The nutrient works as an antidote to that dismal companion of pain, depression, whose amelioration is almost always associated with pain reduction. Following Dr. Ehrenpreis's lead, clinical investigators identified several other nutrient antidepressants that contribute to the control of pain.

The antidepressant/pain-control nutrient that Dr. Ehrenpreis discovered is DLPA (DL-*p*henyl*a*lanine), which is found in such ordinary foods as fish, poultry, vegetables, fruits, and grains. Phenylalanine is one of the twenty-two amino acids that are the building blocks of all living things. Occurring in nature in two forms, D and L, which are the mirror images of each other, phenylalanine is available in pharmacies and health food stores as a food supplement containing both forms in a fifty-fifty mixture.

The other antidepressant nutrients helpful in controlling pain are two other amino acids and three B-complex vitamins. The amino acids are tyrosine and tryptophan, and the vitamins are $B_3$ (niacin), $B_6$ (pyridoxine), and inositol. Vitamins $B_3$ and $B_6$ are necessary for the metabolism of the antidepressant/pain-control amino acids; and inositol may be relaxing agent, an aid in curbing some depressive states.

In this chapter, you'll become familiar with these nutrients: what they are, what they can do for you, how they work, what to watch for when you use them, what foods are rich in them, and the right supplement dosages for safe and effective relief of pain and depression in a total pain-control program.

# DLPA

## What DLPA Has Done for Others

Claims have been made that DLPA can provide good to excellent relief in as little as two days from low back and postoperative pain, as well as the pain of whiplash, arthritis, and fibrositis of the muscle. Even the agony of cancer is reportedly alleviated by this nutrient.

But these results have not as yet been verified by double-blind studies, medical science's ultimate test of the effectiveness of a therapy. (In a double-blind study, neither the subjects nor the investigators know who is receiving the therapeutic and who is receiving the placebo, a nontherapeutic substance such as water.)

DLPA as an analgesic, therefore, has not entered the mainstream of pain-control therapy. But because of impressive results in double-blind tests, it has been accepted as an antidepressant, when used in conjunction with the tricyclic antidepressant drug imipramine. Major brand names of this drug are Tofranil and Tofranil-PM.

This nutrient-drug combination, said to manage depression successfully in up to nine cases out of ten, contributes to the relief of pain in a total pain-control program.

## What We've Learned About DLPA
## at the Pain Alleviation Center

Antidepressant drugs are, as they are in all major pain-control centers, sometimes an indispensable part of our program. While there are some adverse side effects to these drugs, as there are to all drugs, they can be well tolerated, and antidepressant drugs do have a beneficial influence on the management of pain. They are also one of the means by which patients are helped to break away from narcotic analgesic drugs, which can be ineffective and harmful for some people who use them over extended periods.

So we are happy to report that DLPA does, by and large, enhance the performance of imipramine-type antidepressants. Because of the consequent effect on the alleviation of pain, DLPA has become a useful element in our total pain-control program, and should be in yours.

### *How DLPA Works*

Two of your neurotransmitters, NE (norepinephrine) and DA (dopamine), when they're present in your brain in sufficient quantities, make you feel high; a dearth of them makes you feel low—a type of depression. DLPA is the raw material from which both those neurotransmitters are manufactured in the brain.

When you increase your intake of dietary and supplementary DLPA, according to modern medical theory, you boost your brain's production of NE and DA. Taking an antidepressant tricyclic drug, at the same time decreases the breakdown of those high-inducing neurotransmitters by the brain's nerve cells. Depression is reversed, and that, in turn, may stimulate the flow of your endorphins.

There is some evidence as well, mainly adduced by Dr. Ehrenpreis, that DLPA inhibits the action of substances in the brain that scavenge—literally "chew up"—endorphins before they can become active. This endorphin-protection action may explain why DLPA apparently improves the performance of some analgesics and other kinds of antipain therapies. DLPA in conjunction with aspirin or acupuncture, for example, has been reported to provide greater pain relief than any of those treatments alone.

### How to Get the Right Amount of DLPA in Your Pain-Control Program

Diet supplies the average American adult with about 2,800 milligrams (approximately one tenth of an ounce) of DLPA daily. That's more than the about 2,200 milligrams set by Dr. William Rose of the University of Illinois as optimal for human health. Presumably, then, most adult Americans are consuming sufficient DLPA in their foods to help ward off chronic pain and depression.

But for the millions of Americans who suffer from those twin afflictions, 2,800 milligrams a day appear to offer no protection. Patients have been known to consume about 5,000 milligrams of DLPA in their daily meals—about twice the national average—and still suffer from chronic pain and depression.

Since it's difficult to obtain more than 5,000 milligrams a day from food, pain-control specialists, following Dr. Ehrenpreis's lead, have augmented their patients' diets with DLPA supplements. At the Pain Alleviation Center, these are combined with a DLPA-rich diet to meet the special high DLPA requirements of chronic-pain sufferers.

## INSTRUCTIONS FOR USING DLPA

1. Be certain that DLPA-rich foods are part of your daily diet by following the Pain-Control Menu Plan (page 107). (A list of the ten best DLPA foods appears on page 96.)

2. Start by taking 1,000 milligrams four times a day—with meals and before bedtime. DLPA supplements are available at pharmacies and health food stores. No prescription is necessary.

3. If there's no improvement in your condition, after two weeks add 500 milligrams of DLPA four times a day. Continue until your pain and depression symptoms are markedly relieved and for one week afterward. Then reduce the amount of DLPA you take by 1,000 milligrams a day. If on any day your symptoms return, restore the previous day's dosage. That's your "threshold dosage" below which DLPA is ineffective. Some patients may have to continue on a threshold dosage for life. Others may gradually reduce their dosage to zero without adverse effects.

4. Be certain to take the vitamin supplements recommended in the Pain-Control Menu Plan. DLPA cannot be converted in the brain to the depression-fighting neurotransmitters NE and DA without ample quantities of vitamins C (ascorbic acid) and $B_6$ (pyridoxine).

### What to Watch For

1. If you think that because some DLPA is good, more would be better, you're wrong. Overdoses may induce insomnia, irritability, headaches, and a new character trait that could get you in trouble: belligerence. Stay with the prescribed doses; if any of those side effects show up, cut back.

2. If you have high blood pressure, consult your supervising doctor about dosages. He or she will probably suggest that even if you don't have high blood pressure, your blood pressure should be monitored while you are on DLPA because it has been known to raise blood pressure in some susceptible

individuals. If that should happen, your doctor will probably suggest a lower dosage.

3. If you're on an antidepressant of the MAO (Monamine oxidase)-inhibitor class, do not take DLPA without your doctor's permission. The combination could raise the blood pressure of susceptible individuals to dangerous levels. MAO-inhibitors include Eutonyl, Marplan, Nardil, and Parnate.

4. If you're pregnant or breast-feeding, do not take DLPA. In cases of phenylketonuria, a genetic disease that may attack your unborn child or infant without your being aware of it, DLPA and its breakdown products can destroy brain tissue, possibly leading to retardation.

5. If you are a victim of pigmented melanoma, do not take DLPA. A melanoma is a mole colored with the dark pigment melanin found in and skin and hair. DLPA can nurture the growth of malignant melanomas, which are a deadly form of skin cancer.

## THE TEN BEST FOOD SOURCES OF DLPA
### (DL-Phenylalanine)

|  | *DLPA Milligrams* |
|---|---|
| Peanuts, shelled, ¾ cup | 1,681 |
| Peanut butter, 6 tablespoons | 1,557 |
| Turkey, 3 ounces cooked | 1,097 |
| Liver, calf's, 3 ounces cooked | 1,095 |
| Chicken, fryer, 3 ounces cooked | 927 |
| Beef, round, 3 ounces cooked | 916 |
| Veal, round, 3 ounces cooked | 905 |
| Lamb, leg, 3 ounces cooked | 837 |
| Halibut, 3 ounces cooked | 789 |
| Cheddar cheese, 3 ounces | 786 |

Other good sources of DLPA include meat, fish, poultry, cottage cheese, soybeans, baked beans, and almonds.

# OTHER NUTRIENTS THAT
# FIGHT PAIN

## Tyrosine

Like DLPA, Tyrosine, an essential amino acid, is converted in the brain into the depression-fighting neurotransmitters NE and DA. In clinical studies, tyrosine supplements have been successful in treating symptoms of depression, sometimes even when other therapies had failed. In one such study, two long-term depressed patients, who had not responded to antidepressant drugs or electroconvulsive shock treatments, were depression-free after the administration of tyrosine.

Tyrosine is so closely related chemically to DLPA that it exhibits many of the same side effects, with these additional two: in susceptible individuals, blood pressure can be dangerously lowered as well as elevated, and migraine may be induced. Because healthful amounts of tyrosine can be obtained in food, and because additional amounts to fight depression are manufactured in the brain from DLPA, tyrosine supplements are not prescribed in your pain-control program.

---

### INSTRUCTIONS FOR USING TYROSINE

1. Be certain that DLPA-rich foods are part of your daily diet by following the Pain-Control Menu Plan (page 107). (A list of the ten best tyrosine foods appears on page 98.)
2. Be certain to take the vitamin supplements recommended in your pain-control program (page 113). Tyrosine cannot be converted in the brain to depression-fighting NE and DA without ample quantities of vitamins C (ascorbic acid) and $B_6$ (pyridoxine).

---

## THE TEN BEST FOOD SOURCES OF TYROSINE

|  | *Tyrosine Milligrams* |
|---|---|
| Peanuts, shelled, ¾ cup | 1,192 |
| Peanut butter, 6 tablespoons | 1,127 |
| Eggs, 2 large | 1,102 |
| Chicken, fryer, 3 ounces cooked | 829 |
| Liver, calf's, 3 ounces cooked | 812 |
| Veal, round, 3 ounces cooked | 802 |
| Beef, round, 3 ounces cooked | 755 |
| Ham, 3 ounces cooked | 745 |
| Lamb, leg, 3 ounces cooked | 714 |
| Halibut, 3 ounces cooked | 574 |

Other good sources of tyrosine include meat, fish, poultry, cottage cheese, soybeans, baked beans, and almonds. Excellent sources are cheese, beer, wine, yeast, ripe bananas, avocados, pickled herring, and chicken liver. However, tyrosine from those sources may bring on or intensify migraine in susceptible individuals.

### L-Tryptophan

Another essential amino acid, L-tryptophan also effectively helps relieve pain by fighting the depression accompanying it. In the presence of ample quantities of $B_3$ (niacin) and $B_6$ (pyridoxine), L-tryptophan, from your diet and as a supplement, is converted in your brain to a natural antidepressant, serotonin. This neurotransmitter produces a feeling of relaxation, security, and serenity.

At the Pain Alleviation Center, we have found L-tryptophan to be most useful as an antidepressant—with consequent analgesic action—when used in conjunction with DLPA and antidepressant drugs. We have also found this nutrient valuable in bringing sleep to insomniacs and helping relieve stress—both pain-abating attributes. Overall, L-tryptophan has been reliably helpful in assuaging moderate pain, particularly in cases of migraine, in a total pain-control program.

L-tryptophan requirements for healthy adults (3 milligrams daily for every 2.2 pounds of body weight, according to the National Academy of Sciences) are met by most Americans from the foods they eat. But chronic-pain sufferers respond only to much larger amounts. While a healthy 150-pounder, for example, needs about 200 milligrams of L-tryptophan a day, a chronic-pain victim of the same weight requires 3,000 or more milligrams to help eliminate pain. These large quantities can be obtained only with the aid of supplements.

---

### INSTRUCTIONS FOR USING L-TRYPTOPHAN

1. Make certain that L-tryptophan-rich foods are part of your daily diet by following the Pain-Control Menu Plan (page 107). (A list of the ten best L-tryptophan foods appears on page 100.)
2. To treat chronic pain and depression, start by taking 500 milligrams of L-tryptophan 4 times a day, at meals and bedtime. L-tryptophan supplements are available at pharmacies and health food stores. No prescription is necessary.
3. After 1 week, raise the bedtime dose to 1,500 milligrams. If there's no significant improvement in your condition after another 2 weeks, add another 500 milligrams before going to sleep.
4. Continue the effective dosage until your pain and depression symptoms are markedly relieved or disappear. After four weeks of relief you can reduce the daily dosage by 500 milligrams for one week. If you are still doing well, reduce the daily dosage another 500 milligrams each week. Should pain

and depression reappear, resume taking the prior week's dosage.

5. To treat insomnia, take an additional 2,000 milligrams with skim milk at bedtime. If that is ineffective, increase the dosage by 1,000 milligrams; if that is still ineffective, add another 1,000 milligrams.

6. Be certain to take the vitamin supplements recommended in the Pain-Control Menu Plan. L-tryptophan cannot be converted in the brain to the depression/insomnia-fighting neurotransmitter serotonin without ample quantities of vitamins $B_3$ (niacin) and $B_6$ (pyridoxine).

### What to Watch For

1. If you experience any of the following possible adverse side effects, discontinue the L-tryptophan supplements and consult the physician who is overseeing your pain-control program:

• Increased fatigue and resistance to activity

• Runny or stuffed nose or congested sinuses

• Intestinal cramps or constipation (a rare side effect)

• Extreme nervousness (a very rare side effect)

2. Because there have recently been unconfirmed reports of injurious effects of tryptophan on the liver, ask your physician's advice about monitoring your liver functions.

## THE TEN BEST FOOD SOURCES OF L-TRYPTOPHAN

|  | *L-Tryptophan Milligrams* |
|---|---|
| Eggs, 2 large | 422 |
| Peanuts, shelled, ¾ cup | 367 |

| | |
|---|---|
| Peanut butter, 6 tablespoons | 336 |
| Liver, calf's, 3 ounces cooked | 327 |
| Veal, round, 3 ounces cooked | 292 |
| Chicken, fryer, 3 ounces | 286 |
| Cheddar cheese, 3 ounces | 270 |
| Lamb, leg, 3 ounces cooked | 266 |
| Beef, round, 3 ounces cooked | 260 |
| Halibut, 3 ounces cooked | 211 |

Other good sources of L-tryptophan include meat, fish, poultry, cheese, soybeans, and milk.

## The Antidepression/Pain Vitamins

The B-complex vitamins: $B_3$, $B_6$, and inositol are the three that have been used effectively as part of the comprehensive pain-control program at the Pain Alleviation Center. They are among the supplements recommended for your pain-control program.

*Vitamin $B_3$* (niacin; sometimes labeled nicotinic acid, niacinamide, or nicotinamide) plays an important role in the brain's production of the antidepression/pain neurotransmitters NE, DA, and serotonin. It is also claimed to have a soothing quality that is helpful in the management of pain. It has been used successfully by some doctors in alleviating the pain of arthritis and to abort the pain of migraine when the headache starts.

*Vitamin $B_6$* (pyridoxine; sometimes labeled pyrodoxal/pyridoxamine) plays a role similar to that of vitamin $B_3$ in the brain's production of antidepression/pain neurotransmitters. This nutrient may also contribute to preventing depletion in the brain of the amino acid gamma-aminobutyric acid (GABA), which acts as a calmative neurotransmitter like serotonin. It is also claimed to strengthen the immune system, which may be hurt by chronic pain.

In addition, *Inositol* (sometimes labeled myoinositol) possibly is an antianxiety, antistress, calming, and relaxing agent, helpful in managing pain.

## INSTRUCTIONS FOR USING VITAMINS
## B₃, B₆, AND INOSITOL

1. Be sure that foods rich in these vitamins are part of your daily diet by following the Pain-Control Menu Plan (page 107). (Lists of the ten best sources of these vitamins appear below.)
2. Be certain to take the vitamin supplements recommended in the Pain-Control Menu Plan. Added to dietary sources, they help provide a safe and healthful level of the three vitamins now associated with pain control.

### *What to Watch For*

1. If you think larger than recommended dosages are better for you, you're wrong. They can be harmful. Dosages indicated in the Pain-Control Menu Plan, added to dietary amounts, provide safe and healthful levels.
2. If you experience any adverse side effects, discontinue taking the vitamins and consult your physician about resuming them on a reduced dosage.

## THE TEN BEST FOOD SOURCES
## FOR EACH VITAMIN
## THAT FIGHTS PAIN AND DEPRESSION

*Basic needs for healthy adults*: $B_3$, 13 to 18 milligrams a day; $B_6$, 2 milligrams a day; inositol 300 to 1,000 milligrams a day. Available from food.

*Safe supplement limits*: $B_3$, 50 to 100 milligrams a day; $B_6$, 50 milligrams a day; inositol, ample quantities are available from food, so no supplementation is necessary. Do not exceed the safe supplement limits without the advice of your doctor.

| $B_3$ (Niacin) | $B_3$ Milligrams |
|---|---|
| Peanuts, shelled, ¾ cup | 18 |
| Liver, 3 ounces cooked | 18 |
| Salmon, 3 ounces cooked | 15 |
| Chicken, 3 ounces cooked | 14 |
| Tuna, 3 ounces cooked | 14 |
| Swordfish, 3 ounces cooked | 13 |
| Turkey, 3 ounces cooked | 13 |
| Rabbit, 3 ounces cooked | 13 |
| Halibut, 3 ounces cooked | 9 |
| Veal, 3 ounces cooked | 8 |

*Other foods that are high in vitamin $B_3$* include lean meats, poultry and fish, brewer's yeast, whole grains, rice bran, and milk and milk products.

| $B_6$ (Pyridoxine) | $B_6$ Milligrams |
|---|---|
| Lentils, 1 cup cooked | 2.6 |
| Sunflower seeds, 1 cup | 1.6 |
| Hazelnuts, shelled, 1 cup | 1.5 |
| Rice, 1 cup cooked | 1.4 |
| Salmon, 3 ounces cooked | 1.1 |
| Wheat germ, 1 cup | 1.0 |
| Tuna, 4 ounces | 1.0 |
| Soybeans, 1 cup cooked | 0.9 |
| Walnuts, shelled, 1 cup | 0.7 |
| Bran, 100% wheat, 1 cup | 0.5 |

*Other foods that are high in vitamin $B_6$* include brewer's yeast, meats, and whole grains.

| Inositol (Myo-inositol) | Inositol Milligrams |
|---|---|
| Grapefruit concentrate, frozen, ½ cup | 456 |
| Wheat germ, ½ cup | 390 |
| Cantaloupe, ¼ average size | 355 |
| Lentils, ¼ cup cooked | 308 |
| Orange, average size | 307 |
| Rice, 1 cup cooked | 298 |

| | |
|---|---|
| Chickpeas (garbanzo beans), ½ cup cooked | 296 |
| Whole wheat bread, 1 slice | 288 |
| Orange concentrate, frozen, ½ cup | 244 |
| Grapefruit, ½ average size | 200 |

*Other foods that are high in inositol* include citrus fruits, brewer's yeast, lean meat, milk, nuts, and vegetables.

# 9

# Your Pain-Control Diet

━━━━━━━━━━

The right diet cannot remit your pain. But it can help in a number of ways.

It can help because it bans those foods that might increase your pain, particularly your headache pain. A roster of them is listed on the following page.

It can help because it includes foods that fight pain-causing degenerative diseases and strengthen the immune system to join in the fight. These foods, which are recommended in the Federal Dietary Guidelines for Americans, are low in fat, saturated fats, and cholesterol.

It can help because it holds to an acceptable minimum the foods that have been indicted, even though not yet convicted, of being injurious to overall body health: sugar and salt.

It can help because it promotes general good health by including foods optimally high in fiber.

It can help because it keeps the calorie content low to bring you to your ideal weight if you're overweight and keep you at your ideal weight if you already are there. Obesity is an ally of poor health—and pain.

It can help because it supplies the right amounts of the right amino acids necessary for the brain to manufacture its quota of painkilling endorphins and antidepressant neurotransmitters.

## FOODS AND SUBSTANCES
## THAT MAY INCREASE YOUR PAIN

| | |
|---|---|
| Alcohol | Hot dogs |
| Avocado | Monosodium glutamate |
| Bacon | (MSG)* |
| Bananas | Nuts |
| Cheese, aged | Pork |
| Chocolate | Red wines |
| Coffee | Sausage |
| Cola drinks | Smoked meats |
| Cold cuts | Tea |
| Fermented foods | Tobacco |
| Herring | Yeast products, fresh baked |

*MSG is present in most Chinese food, meat tenderizers, and preservatives. It is also found in some canned soups, bacon, dry-roasted nuts, frozen dinners, ham, instant gravies, instant soups, processed meats, self-basting turkey, and soy sauce.

It can help because the food is good-tasting as well as nutritious, making it easy for you to make the transition from the foods to which you are accustomed.

## HOW TO USE YOUR
## PAIN-CONTROL DIET

The Pain-Control Menu Plan that begins on page 107 can be followed as it is given, or you can make substitutions each week by replacing any ingredient with a similar ingredient—one kind of fruit for another, for example. Use fresh foods wherever possible.

This is a 1,200 to 1,300 calories-a-day plan, which should help you achieve and maintain your ideal weight. If you're large and need more calories, just increase the portion sizes. But watch your scale and cut back if you find that you are gaining weight.

## The Pain-Control Menu Plan

## DAY 1

### *Breakfast*

1 cup fresh fruit salad
1 scrambled egg cooked in nonstick skillet with 1 teaspoon sweet butter/margarine blend
1 small bran or whole-wheat muffin with 1 teaspoon unsweetened jelly
½ cup low-fat or skim milk
Coffee substitute, fruit juice (no sugar added), or water

### *Lunch*

Medium-sized salad of lettuce and tomatoes with lemon juice
1 broiled lean hamburger on bun
Melon wedge (medium-sized)
Coffee substitute, fruit juice (no sugar added), or water

### *Dinner*

Green salad with up to 2 tablespoons low-calorie, low-sodium salad dressing
5 medium broiled shrimp (about 4 ounces)
1 small baked potato with dollop of low-fat plain yogurt and minced fresh herbs or green onion (eat potato skin)
1 small baked apple, sweetened with 1 teaspoon honey
½ cup low-fat or skim milk
Coffee substitute, fruit juice (no sugar added), or water

# DAY 2

### Breakfast

1 orange
½ cup hot oatmeal or Wheatena sweetened with apple juice
  (no sugar added), sprinkled with 2 teaspoons plain
  toasted wheat germ
½ cup low-fat or skim milk
Coffee substitute, fruit juice (no sugar added), or water

### Lunch

1 cup low-sodium consommé
Salad of cucumbers, green peppers, bean sprouts, and wa-
  tercress with lemon juice
Open-face sandwich of 1 ounce Jarlsberg cheese on whole-
  wheat bread
Herb tea or club soda with lime

### Dinner

1 cup tomato juice (no salt added)
Medium-sized mixed green salad with grated carrot with up
  to 2 tablespoons low-calorie, low-sodium salad dressing
3 ounces sliced roast chicken (without skin)
Steamed asparagus, broccoli, or cauliflower (medium
  portion)
½ cup cubed fresh pineapple or canned pineapple in its own
  juice
½ cup low-fat or skim milk
Coffee substitute, fruit juice (no sugar added), or water

# DAY 3

### Breakfast

1 cup melon balls
Western omelet, consisting of 1 egg yolk, 2 egg whites, and

herb/spice seasonings, filled with sautéed sweet peppers, onions, and tomatoes, cooked in nonstick skillet with one teaspoon sweet butter/margarine blend
1 slice whole-wheat toast with 1 teaspoon honey or unsweet-ened jelly
1 cup low-fat or skim milk
Coffee substitute, fruit juice (no sugar added), or water

### Lunch

Salad of lettuce, tomatoes, watercress, and 4 boiled or broiled shrimp with lemon juice
1 slice whole-wheat bread
1 cup fresh fruit salad
Herb tea or club soda with lime

### Dinner

Mixed green salad with up to 2 tablespoons low-calorie, low-sodium salad dressing
4 ounces well-trimmed broiled sirloin steak with sliced onions
½ cup steamed fresh peas or carrots
1-inch-slice angel food cake
½ cup low-fat or skim milk
Coffee substitute, fruit juice (no sugar added), or water

# DAY 4

### Breakfast

1 orange
1 shredded Wheat biscuit sprinkled with 1 teaspoon date powder (available in health food stores)
½ cup low-fat or skim milk
Coffee substitute, fruit juice (no sugar added), or water

## *Lunch*

Salad of shredded carrots, cabbage, and sweet green peppers
    with lemon juice
3 ounces sliced turkey (not turkey roll) or chicken (without
    skin)
1 slice whole-wheat bread
Melon wedge
Herb tea or club soda with lime

## *Dinner*

Salad of shredded zucchini, sliced tomatoes, watercress, and
    sweet peppers with up to 2 tablespoons low-calorie, low-
    sodium salad dressing
4 ounces broiled fillet of sole
Steamed asparagus, broccoli, cauliflower, or green beans
1 piece fresh fruit
1 cup low-fat or skim milk
Coffee substitute, fruit juice (no sugar added), or water

# DAY 5

## *Breakfast*

4 stewed prunes
1 small bran or whole-wheat muffin with 2 tablespoons low-
    fat cottage cheese
1 cup low-fat or skim milk
Coffee substitute, fruit juice (no sugar added), or water

## *Lunch*

Lettuce and tomato salad with up to 2 tablespoons low-cal-
    orie, low-sodium salad dressing
1 cup low-sodium vegetable or minestrone soup

Open-face sandwich of 1 ounce Jarlsberg cheese on whole-wheat bread
1 cup fresh fruit salad
Herb tea or club soda with lime

### Dinner

Salad of chicory, endive, bean sprouts, and tomatoes with lemon juice
2 small, well-trimmed broiled lamb chops or 1 medium broiled veal chop
½ cup steamed carrots
1-inch-slice angel food cake
½ cup low-fat or skim milk
Coffee substitute, fruit juice (no sugar added), or water

## DAY 6

### Breakfast

½ grapefruit sweetened with 1 spoonful honey and sprinkled with 2 teaspoons plain toasted wheat germ
1 slice French toast prepared in nonstick skillet with 1 egg, 1 teaspoon sweet butter/margarine blend, sprinkled with cinnamon
½ cup low-fat or skim milk
Coffee substitute, fruit juice (no sugar added), or water

### Lunch

Mixed green salad with bean sprouts and up to 2 tablespoons low-calorie, low-sodium salad dressing
Open-face sandwich of canned water-packed tuna or salmon (no salt added), sprinkled with lemon juice, on whole-wheat bread
Melon wedge
Herb tea or club soda with lime

## Dinner

1 cup tomato juice (no salt added)
Salad of sliced cucumbers, radishes, watercress, and tomatoes with lemon juice
3 ounces sliced broiled or roast chicken (without skin)
½ cup steamed Brussels sprouts, broccoli, or turnips
1 piece fresh fruit
½ cup low-fat or skim milk
Coffee substitute, fruit juice (no sugar added), or water

# DAY 7

## Breakfast

½ cup hot cereal of your choice sweetened with apple juice (no sugar added) and cinnamon
1 slice whole-wheat toast with 1 teaspoon sweet butter/margarine blend and 1 teaspoon unsweetened jelly
1 cup low-fat or skim milk
Coffee substitute, fruit juice (no sugar added), or water

## Lunch

Chef's salad consisting of tomatoes, spinach leaves, cucumbers, radishes, and 3 ounces cubed chicken or turkey (not turkey roll) with up to 2 tablespoons low-calorie, low-sodium salad dressing
1 small baked apple sweetened with 1 teaspoon honey and sprinkled with 1 teaspoon date powder (available in health food stores)
Herb tea or club soda with lime

## Dinner

1 cup of low-sodium consommé
Mixed green salad with tomatoes, watercress, and cucumbers

4 ounces broiled or baked salmon or swordfish
½ cup steamed green beans
1 small baked potato with dollop of low-fat plain yogurt and
    minced fresh herbs or green onion (eat potato skin)
1 cup diced fresh fruit (grapefruit, orange, melon, berries)
½ cup low-fat or skim milk
Coffee substitute, fruit juice (no sugar added), or water

## SHOULD YOU TAKE
## VITAMIN/MINERAL SUPPLEMENTS?

Yes. A one-a-day multiple vitamin/mineral supplement can help replace these vital substances that you may lose as a result of your condition. Optimal amounts of vitamins and minerals are necessary not only for general health but also for the manufacture of endorphins and neurotransmitters. Take your supplement with one of your meals, preferably breakfast.

# 10

# The Pain Capsule: A New Way to Break Drug Dependency

If you're a victim of chronic benign pain (not the pain of cancer), the various techniques of your pain-control program could replace narcotic analgesic drugs and sedative hypnotics. (A list of popularly prescribed drugs in these categories appears on pages 122–25.) At the Pain Alleviation Center, we have found that almost all chronic benign pain patients are better off without these drugs, and our study of the scientific literature has reinforced our findings.

Patients taking these drugs (abbreviated hereafter as A/S drugs), experience these undesirable effects:

- At first, sleeplessness after taking sleeping pills for some time, and a consequent upping of sleeping pill dosage
- Then, a mild anxiety, a vague restlessness, often masked by the pain, with the overall effect of the pain's worsening
- Later, the risk of addiction, producing a strain between the doctor who wants to withhold the medication and the patient who craves it
- The growing desire for the drugs clashing with the patient's will to avoid dangerous overdosing—a tension heightened in

> hours-long waits in misery until the patient "can't take it any-
> more" and "pops" the pills before due time
- Finally, the sad realization that A/S drugs actually perpetuate
  chronic pain instead of helping to relieve it
- By this time, the patient is drug-dependent, and sudden withdrawal is certain to produce pernicious symptoms.

## BREAKING THE A/S DRUG HABIT

In 1983, heading a team of medical pain-control specialists at the
Pain Alleviation Center, I conducted a study of a new method we
had developed for breaking the A/S drug habit. It is a safe way that
can be carried out without any effort by the patient and without
tension. In a paper on that study presented before the American
Pain Society, I described this innovative method and presented the
results of its application.

The title of the paper was *Use of a Pain Capsule to Eliminate
Drug Intake of Chronic-Pain Patients in an Outpatient Treatment
Center.* What follows are excerpts from an abstract of that paper,
with my comments.

I first pinpointed the problem: "Patients with benign chronic
pain are frequently prescribed drugs on a pain-contingent basis
(prn)." That is, the drugs are to be taken as needed. There's
a danger here, because prn "sometimes results in iatrogenic
drug dependence"—doctor-induced addiction to a therapeutic
drug.

Our task was to solve the problem by eliminating the drug dependence with no harm to the patient, which meant two things:
first, no intensification of pain, which could be managed through
our regimen of new pain therapies that actually lessen the pain,
with which you are already familiar, and second, no withdrawal
symptoms.

I knew, as all doctors know, how dangerous it is to suddenly
stop taking A/S medications, particularly narcotic analgesics. Un-
used to being without medication, your body may feel increased
pain. In worse cases, the craving for the drug is overpowering. You

get the shakes, your heart races, you can't be still for a moment, you're in panic. You feel your body in violent rebellion. You're assailed by stomach cramps and nausea, chills and sweating, muscle pains. You wear the sign of the drug addict in withdrawal: the wide, staring pupils of your eyes.

I proposed an "approach to eliminate this drug dependence [by] having patients on a regular timed schedule, and *gradually reducing the active ingredients.*" Correct in theory, my research team agreed, but not workable in practice. If the patients knew when the dosage was being decreased, and by how much, it would cause an emotional storm. Dependent, they needed the drug; they needed it at the strength they were used to; and they needed it at that strength all the time. But if they didn't know when the dosage was being decreased and by how much, how could they tell the difference? Ignorance would be bliss as long as we reduced the dose slowly enough to avoid withdrawal problems.

This is how I arranged the details.

"With the consent of the patients, we made arrangements with their pharmacists to combine all their prescribed pain medications into individualized standardized capsules." Now the patient had only a single capsule to take. "All capsules were self-administered on a time-contingent schedule." The patients took the capsules, not prn, but at fixed times. Our patients had no objection to doing this, feeling, and rightly so, that their daily dosage would manage their pain as well as the former prn dosage.

"Over periods of one to three months, the active ingredients in the capsules were gradually reduced on a schedule unknown by the patients." This was done with the collaboration of the pharmacist. A copy of my letter of instructions to the pharmacists appears on pages 118–19. You should read it because it fleshes out the details of the capsules' preparation and use, and why they're necessary.

With no knowledge of the dosage reductions, the patients in our study showed no adverse psychological reactions. It is possible that, as the reductions occurred, the placebo effect took over, and the patients' own brains were producing more endorphins to hold back the pain. At the same time, our new nondrug therapies were certainly boosting endorphin production. As the amounts of A/S drugs in the capsules gradually declined, the patients steadily improved.

Dear Pharmacist:

Thank you for agreeing to cooperate with us on using our "pain capsule regimen" for patient Joe Jones [Jane Smith].

While we realize the compounding of the "pain capsule" requires extra time and effort on your part, we feel certain that this will ultimately benefit the patient greatly.

As I mentioned during our phone conversation, our patient has been taking narcotic analgesics and/or sedative hypnotics on a prn basis for quite some time. We have found that this method of taking these medications serves to reinforce the chronic-pain syndrome and, if anything, serves to perpetuate and worsen the patient's problem.

Our ultimate goal is to reduce and eventually eliminate all narcotic analgesics and/or sedative hypnotics in this patient, but we feel the best way to go about it is, first, to substitute a time schedule of medication intake for the prn schedule. This will help the patient not to focus on "the pill" as the answer to his [her] pain problem. He [She] will then be able to utilize our non-pharmacologic pain-control methods such as biofeedback, self-hypnosis, etc., and begin to focus in on these instead of the pills.

In addition, placing the medication in an unmarked capsule will reduce the external clues to the patient that we are reducing the medication. Although the patient knows that our ultimate goal is to gradually reduce the medication, he [she] will not be aware of when and by how much we are making these reductions. It is for this reason that the external appearance of the capsule must be similar from week to week.

The patient has been instructed not to ask our staff or yours for information about the contents or the amount of the medication. In fact, the medication in the capsules at first is usually the identical medication that the patient was taking at the time of his [her] initial evaluation at our center.

We would further appreciate it if the costs of the prescription and compounding could be averaged over the entire period of time for which the medication will be prescribed and that the costs remain the same from week to week. This will, again, avoid giving the patient clues that the medication is being reduced.

Finally, if for any reason the patient does not pick up the medication for the week, please contact our office and let us know immediately, or when we call in the following week's prescription. If there are any other problems either with the patient or the medication, please contact us.

I want to thank you again for your cooperation and to encourage you to call this office if you have any questions or if there is any difficulty with this program.

Sincerely,
Richard M. Linchitz, M.D.
Medical Director
Pain Alleviation Center

---

The results of our study showed that "of the 21 patients placed on the pain-pill regimen, complete elimination [of the A/S drugs] was accomplished by 12. Of the nine patients who did not completely eliminate their medications during treatment, three later became drug-free."

Could these people remain off pain-control drugs? Two years after the study, half of the patients who were off drugs had stayed off drugs. Since the study was made in 1983, the stay-off success record of the pain-capsule regimen has soared. About 75 percent of our chronic-benign-pain patients have, through 1987, eliminated A/S drugs.

"These results suggest," I concluded, "that a pain-capsule regimen can be effective in eliminating reliance upon pain medications of chronic-pain patients being treated *in an outpatient setting.*"

As, in essence, you are.

# HOW YOU CAN USE
# THE PAIN-CAPSULE REGIMEN

The physician overseeing your pain-control program can write a letter similar to mine to your pharmacist after a preliminary phone call. Like the outpatients at the Pain Alleviation Center, you'll know that your medication is going to be cut down, but you won't know when and by how much. There will be no psychological upheaval. But—and this is mandatory—during the course of the pain-capsule regimen do adhere rigorously to your program of nondrug therapies. If you are like most of the chronic-benign patients at the Pain Alleviation Center, you will experience less pain as your drug dosage is lessened, and far less pain when you reach "Drug dosage: Zero."

Why, you may ask, as many of our patients have, did doctors prescribe these drugs in the first place? Because your doctor's goal is to provide you with some relief from your suffering. A/S drug-free means of pain control such as those of your pain-control program have not been available up to now for the majority of chronic-pain patients. It is likely that, in the future, your doctor may suggest such a program or refer you to a pain-control center that offers one.

But, face it—you are as responsible as your doctor for drug therapy. Like most patients brought up in a society in which pill-popping is a way of life, it's natural for you to demand pills as a quick fix for your pain. Until you had considered the treatment described in this book, and until you had proved to yourself that nondrug therapy *can* work, you probably would not commit yourself to the tough work of ridding yourself of pain without A/S drugs. You would continue to demand a pill, and if your doctor didn't give it to you, you might change doctors.

*That's* another reason your doctor writes prescriptions for you, why doctors in this country write 24 billion prescriptions a year—the number is so huge that it's unfathomable. Tell your doctor that you want a chronic-pain treatment which does not depend mainly on drugs, and your doctor will almost surely cooperate.

## WHEN DRUGS ARE RIGHT FOR YOU

In chronic non-benign pain—the pain, for example, of advanced cancer—concerns about A/S-drug drawbacks pale before the urgency of treating the disease itself and making the patient as comfortable as possible. Even when a nondrug chronic-pain program for a nonthreatening disease is planned, doctors often prescribe A/S drugs at first. The doctors' initial response, to alleviate the pain at once, is the right response.

As a matter of fact, A/S drugs are sometimes underused. I have in mind cases of the chronic cancer pain. The proper schedule for administering drugs (fixed times as opposed to prn) can be helpful, as can the use of other medications—"pain modulators"—to boost the effect of the A/S drugs. In many cases, antidepressant drugs are recommended, especially in combination with the nutrient supplements DLPA and L-tryptophan.

How you can best use A/S and other drugs and which are the best ones to use are matters for you to discuss with the physician overseeing your pain-control program.

## A CHRONIC-PAIN SUFFERER'S GUIDE TO THERAPEUTIC DRUGS

Drugs are potent weapons in medicine's ongoing battle against illness, mental as well as physical. Without drugs untold numbers of lives would terminate prematurely, sicknesses by the millions would linger unendurably, and the population of the emotionally disturbed would explode exponentially.

But drugs aren't panaceas. They aren't miracles in a capsule. There is no drug that has no adverse side effect, ranging from feeble to fatal. There is no drug that isn't a mixture of the good and the bad. But, by and large, the good outweighs the bad, and that means help for you.

You should know about this balance between the good and the bad in drugs, because drugs are usually the first weapons mobilized in your fight against pain—the first hope, which may appear to you as the only hope—and should that hope be placed in jeopardy by the bad, you may lose all hope. The bad in drugs is part of the drugs, but so is the good—and that's the part that counts. The only drugs we do not recommend are A/S drugs when used over long periods in cases of chronic benign pain.

The following are the most commonly prescribed pain-control drugs, sedatives, and antidepressants.

## Pain-control Drugs

These drugs are identified as narcotic or non-narcotic. Narcotic analgesics, ordinarily stronger than non-narcotic analgesics, are derived from potent mind-altering drugs, some of which, including morphine, are members of the opium family. Non-narcotic analgesics are based on other chemical formulations that have minor or no mind-altering properties. As a rule of thumb, narcotic analgesics can be addictive; non-narcotic drugs cannot, even though psychological dependency may result from extended use.

### *Acetaminophen*

Non-narcotic, mild. Reduces fever as well as pain. Common side effects: possible drowsiness; with mild overdose, irritability. Nonprescription.

### *Aspirin (Sodium Salicylate)*

Non-narcotic, mild. Reduces fever and inflammation as well as pain. Common side effects: ringing in ears, nausea, vomiting, abdominal pain, stomach upset, heartburn, and indigestion in susceptible individuals. Nonprescription.

### *Codeine*

Narcotic, mild. Common side effects: nausea, constipation, dizziness, flushed face, difficulty in urination, fatigue; dulls alertness and reflexes. Prescription.

### *Darvon (Propoxyphene)*

Narcotic, mild. Similar to codeine, but less likely to induce nausea and constipation and may cause stomach upset. Prescription.

### *Demerol (Meperidine)*

Narcotic, strong. See *Codeine.* Prescription. Potentially very addictive.

### *Dilaudid (Hydromorphone)*

Narcotic, very strong. Produces a powerful high. See *Codeine.* Side effects accentuated when dosages are increased to maintain initial high and painkilling effect, at which time vomiting and loss of mental alertness is likely to occur. Prescription. Potentially very addictive.

### *Morphine*

Narcotic, very strong. See *Dilaudid.* Prescription. Potentially very addictive.

### *Percodan*

Contains a strong narcotic (oxycodone) and aspirin, strong. See *Codeine.* Prescription. Potentially very addictive.

### *Tylenol*

Non-narcotic, mild. See *Acetominophen.* Nonprescription.

## Antidepressant Drugs

### *Elavil (Amitriptyline)*

A tricyclic antidepressant, effective in two to three weeks, most effective in eight. Common side effects for susceptible individuals:

headache, insomnia, dry mouth, unpleasant taste, constipation or diarrhea, nausea, indigestion, craving for sugar, fatigue, weakness. Most patients, however, can cope with side effects, which generally do not occur in clusters and are mild. Prescription.

### Marplan

MAO (monamine oxidase) inhibitor. Effective in two to three weeks, most effective in six. Common side effects for susceptible individuals: dizziness, constipation, difficulties in urination, fatigue, and weakness. Most patients, however, can cope with side effects, which generally do not occur in clusters and are mild. Prescription.

### Nardil

See *Marplan.*

### Parnate

See *Marplan.*

### Tofranil (Imipramine)

See *Elavil.*

## Sedatives (Tranquilizers)

### Butisol

Barbiturate. Addictive after prolonged use. Common side effects: dizziness, drowsiness, feeling of hangover. In treatment of sleep disorders, rapidly becomes ineffective. Symptoms of anxiety may develop after extended use. Prescription. Potentially very addictive.

### Librium (Chlordiazepoxide)

See *Valium.* Potentially very addictive.

### Luminal

See *Butisol.* Potentially very addictive.

### Nembutal

See *Butisol.* Potentially very addictive.

### Seconal

See *Butisol.* Potentially very addictive.

### Tuinal

See *Butisol.*

### Valium (Diazepam)

Effective in two hours for pain-associated problems of anxiety, tension, and muscle spasm. Common side effects: clumsiness, drowsiness, dizziness; after use over an extended period: nausea, constipation, blurred vision, and increased depression. Prescription. Potentially very addictive.

# 11

# Changing Your and Your Family's Attitudes Toward Your Pain

Chronic pain can so alter your psychological profile that the former you and the present you bear little resemblance to each other. The you in pain—if you're like millions on millions of chronic sufferers for whom pain is a day-in, day-out ordeal that cripples their lives—perversely perpetuates your pain and in the fallout alienates your family. The you in pain is your enemy and that of your family.

For your own sake and for your family's sake, you have to change—not back to your old self, but to a better self. You have to become your own best friend. You also have to become your family's best friend, not the stranger pain has made you. You have to accept for yourself the ultimate responsibility of loving and being loved, because only then can you create an emotional force powerful enough to erase the psychological profile of the you in pain.

It can be done. Others have done it. "I am not responsible for my illness," one mother of three told me. "But I am responsible for myself. I am responsible for my family. I am responsible for making myself well. I will not let negative attitudes crush these responsibilities. I will change."

She did. First, as you should do, by checking whether her psychological profile matches the psychological profile of most chronic-pain sufferers. It did. Yours will probably match it as well. If it does, then, as this mother did, follow the advice of psychological, social, spiritual, and marital counselors, distilled here for you, for creating a new psychological profile of yourself.

It is that new profile of you, helping defeat your pain, that will change your attitude, and consequently your family's attitude, to your pain.

## CHANGING YOUR ATTITUDE TOWARD YOUR PAIN

The psychological pain profile that follows is a composite of that of the many thousands of patients treated by pain-control specialists and pain-control centers throughout the nation, including the Pain Alleviation Center. It is made up of psychological units—hopelessness, for example—that you are apt to share with most of your fellow chronic-pain sufferers. *As you read them, note the ones that afflict you, then practice the suggested remedy.*

Remember, the you in pain is not your fault. But if you don't try to change to a better you, *that* is your fault. Accept this help and act on it. It could help make your fight against pain winnable, and winnable faster. It could make you happier. And when your pain is gone, it could make you a more fulfilled human being.

### *"I feel hopeless and helpless."*

Not now you don't. Count your blessings. Out loud. First thing each day. Look at yourself in the mirror when you recite them and watch your face brighten.

"I am getting better because I exercise."
"I am getting better because I practice relaxation techniques."
"I am getting better because I practice autogenics."
"I am getting better because I practice self-hypnosis."
"I am getting better because I watch the movies of my mind."

"I am getting better because I take DLPA and L-tryptophan supplements."

"I am getting better because I'm sticking to my pain-control diet."

"I am getting better because I'm working on changing my and my family's attitudes to pain."

"I am getting better because I'm off painkilling drugs."

"I am getting better because with all these things working for me, I cannot feel hopeless and helpless."

"I am feeling better because I know I'm helping myself and I have hope."

And add the formula of the French psychologist Emile Coué on a note of firm conviction: "Every day, in every way, I'm getting better and better."

### *"I am depressed."*

Ask yourself, "Why?" You've tried the techniques of your pain-control program, and you've *felt* the results, actually had *proof* of the results in your biofeedback exercises. What's there to be depressed about? Tell yourself all the reasons why you shouldn't feel depressed. Out loud. Do it at noon in front of a mirror. Take a good look at your face. It looks the opposite of depressed.

"I'm not depressed because *now* I sleep well."

"I'm not depressed because *now* I feel good about myself."

"I'm not depressed because *now* I think straight."

"I'm not depressed because *now* I'm active."

"I'm not depressed because *now* I'm interested in things."

"I'm not depressed because *now* I'm seeing my friends."

"I'm not depressed because *now* I'm working on getting along better with my family."

"I'm not depressed because *now* I feel alert—thanks to getting off painkilling drugs."

"I'm not depressed because *now* I don't worry about being depressed."

"I'm not depressed because DLPA and L-tryptophan make me feel 'up.'"

"I'm not depressed because *now* I don't want to be depressed."

And, as you did in the morning, repeat with firm conviction, "Every day, in every way, I'm getting better and better."

### *"I feel my family is not supportive."*

That may be your fault. They want to be, but you won't let them. Mostly, because you ask too much of them emotionally, demand to be waited on hand and foot, insist that the family's purpose is to take care of you. Why? Haven't you learned in all the weeks you've been doing your pain-control program exercises that you can basically take care of yourself? The family will pitch in without resentment, without rancor, only when *you* pitch in. Only when *you* stop using your sickness to push them around. So, if you haven't done so already, resolve to do the following. Make your resolutions out loud, in front of a mirror, and see how much better you like yourself. Before going to bed is a good time.

"I resolve not to use my pain as an excuse to be pampered."

"I resolve not to use my pain as an excuse to be nasty."

"I resolve not to use my pain as an excuse for not taking part in family decisions."

"I resolve not to use my pain as an excuse to turn my family into paramedics."

"I resolve not to use my pain as an excuse to dominate conversations."

"I resolve not to use my pain to get what I want emotionally."

"I resolve not to use my pain to get my family to do what I want them to do."

"I resolve not to take my guilt feelings about being in pain out on the family."

"I resolve not to be mean to my spouse to cover up my loss of interest in sex."

"I resolve not to infect my family with my negative thoughts, but to think positively instead."

"I resolve not to be the picture of misery in front of my family, but to put a good face on things."

And, as you did twice before, sum up with firm conviction, "Every day, in every way, I'm getting better and better."

With these exercises linked to your pain-control program, you can erase the psychological profile of the you in pain—helpless, hopeless, depressed, alienated from your family—and help turn yourself around to a self-helpful person, brimming with hope, becoming part of a happier family.

## CHANGING YOUR FAMILY'S ATTITUDES TOWARD YOUR PAIN

If you carry out your resolutions to gain your family's support, you're on your way. But carry them out. Deeds count.

You can also, with the aid of your supervising physician, point out some ways in which your family members can help you without disabling themselves.

### *Tell Them They Can Help by Becoming Your Cheering Section.*

Tell them that your pain-control program, as excellent as it is, has little or no chance of succeeding without their encouragement. Tell them that you're reaching out for a loving rapport. Won't they reach out to you? They love you, and they will. When they begin to ask, "Seen any good movies of the mind lately?" you'll know they're very much on your side.

### *Tell Them They Can Help by Taking the Focus of Family Life Off Your Illness.*

Tell them that you won't talk about it all the time, and ask them not to. Tell them you won't coerce them into making your pain the center of family life, and ask them to live as if it was just a problem they can all cope with as a matter of course. "Easy does it," tell them. "Let's go on with our lives." They'll like that. They've missed the exchanges of love, of earnest communication, even of sibling rivalries. You'll feel better, too, as part of a real family, not a grim hospital staff.

### Ask Them to Show Their Affection
### When You Feel Good, Not When You Feel Bad.

Tell them that a show of affection when you feel bad seems like a reward for being in pain. Tell them you want a reward for *not* being in pain. When you say, "I feel great today," that's the time for them to applaud, to show their love. You want more of that, and you'll get better faster because of it. The faster you get better, the happier your family will be.

### Ask Them to Try Some
### of Your Pain-Control Techniques for Themselves.

Tell them they will feel as you do, and so empathize with you. Tell them to try total relaxation techniques, especially transcendental meditation. Tell them to start off thinking of it as a game. Then, when they feel that sense of well-being, the smoothing away of stress, they may see it as a valuable asset, a gift you've given them to improve their lives. That draws you and your family closer together. You can even, as some families do, meditate together. Family meditation, according to one study, makes the meditation more effective for you.

### Ask Them to Help You Stay
### on Your Pain-Control Program.

Tell them to check up on you: "Did you take your DLPA?" "Did you do your exercises?" Are you sure you put in the full twenty minutes on your deep breathing?" The sense of affectionate concern lifts your spirits—and that's an aid to beating pain. What's more, it *does* help you stick to your program, on schedule, with no cheating.

### Tell Them You Don't Want Them
### to Be Grim Just Because You're Sick.

Tell them that fun and laughter are wonderful ways to alleviate your pain. Tell them to get rid of their sickroom faces and be themselves. Happiness is contagious, and you'd like to catch some of theirs. Tell them it does wonders for your pain. You're clearing up an oppressive atmosphere, and they'll be delighted to go along with you.

### Ask Them to Share
### Your Pain-Control Diet.

It's as delicious as it is nutritious. Food works fast changes, and in just a few weeks they'll feel better, more vigorous, more alive. You won't feel like an alien at meals. Sharing food is one of the most intimate and binding of all family experiences. That experience can be yours, creating a wave of good feeling three times a day that can help wash away your pain.

### Ask Them to Speak Up
### If They Have Any Complaints About Your Behavior.

If you can change it for the better, do it. If you can't, tell them why. Frank communication dispels resentment, relieves you of that pain-boosting emotional burden, keeps the family content. An atmosphere of contentment helps you cope with pain.

### Ask Them to Tell You
### That They Believe in Your Pain-Control Program.

They've seen it work, they've tried some of it themselves, they *do* believe. Telling that to you has a placebo effect: it stimulates your endorphins, it's a catalyst that speeds your recovery. *Their* belief strengthens *your* belief.

You may find that changing you and your family's attitudes toward your pain is, because of the degree of your pain, too difficult a task. That is when your supervising physician will direct you to the counselor or counselors who can best help you, or help you to help yourself. When you change your and your family's attitudes toward your pain into positive attitudes, you're not fighting alone, you're fighting with an elite corps: your family, fiercely devoted to making you well. You and your family are a pain-fighting unit that can't be beaten. Believe it.

# PART THREE

# PUTTING YOUR CHRONIC-PAIN CONTROL PROGRAM TO WORK

# 12

# Your Hour-by-Hour Chronic-Pain-Control Program

You now should be convinced of the exceptional benefits of your pain-control program. You can relieve your pain. You can break your drug habit. You can become a better you. You can relate to your family, and they can relate to you, in a more loving way. And you should know from your practice sessions that your pain-control program works. You have a powerful group of incentives for going on, and staying on, the program.

The success of your pain-control program depends on you. You must follow it rigorously. Never let a day pass without adhering to it. Never cut out a session. Never cut a session short. Never fail to give every session your all. Never deviate from the pain-control diet. Never let your enthusiasm flag.

Sure, you're going to work and work hard. But reread the foregoing paragraph. The rewards are worth all the effort you put into it.

## YOUR DAILY PROGRAM

Before you begin this program, be sure you have learned each of the new pain-control techniques in the preceding chapters. While you have been learning, be sure you have switched to the pain-control diet and changed you and your family's attitudes to your pain. All this may take two to three months, but in the process you will have improved significantly.

In the following schedule Hour 1 is your normal wake-up time; Hour 2 is an hour later; Hour 3, two hours later; and so forth. For the purpose of clarity, we arbitrarily selected 7:00 A.M. as your wake-up time; that time appears in parenthesis after Hour 1; 8:00 A.M. after Hour 2; 9:00 A.M. after Hour 3; and so forth. The schedule is intended for a person who spends the day at home. It should be reviewed by the physician supervising your pain-control program; he or she may recommend modifications, including alternate or additional therapies, depending on your condition and lifestyle.

### Hour 1 (7:00 A.M.)

Perform your Get-Going Exercises in bed. These gentle stretching exercises relieve muscle tension and stiffness and start the flow of your brain's own painkillers, the endorphins.

Follow your Get-Going Exercises with a twenty-minute total relaxation technique. Transcendental meditation (TM) is preferred by many chronic-pain sufferers.

### Hour 2 (8:00 A.M.)

Breakfast with the whole family. Make the selection from your pain-control diet, or use your own variation. Encourage the whole family to eat what you do, but don't be rigid with them. Get into the conversation, but don't talk about your pain. Take your DLPA, L-tryptophan, and vitamin/mineral supplements.

### Hour 3 (9:00 A.M.)

Do household chores for no longer than fifteen minutes. Perform exercises that relieve tension in your back, neck, and shoulder muscles. View a six-second movie of your mind. After each fifteen minutes of work during the day, repeat the exercises and movie of your mind. About three hours of work are your limit at this stage of your recovery. As you feel better and better, extend your work hours. A hobby requiring physical activity is a fine substitute for work, and a stress reliever, too. This regimen prepares you to go back to your job before too long.

### Hours 4 to 6 (10:00 A.M. to Noon)

Repeat Hour 3, but add a twenty-minute session of autogenics after exercises, then follow with your movie of the mind. Self-hypnosis may be substituted for autogenics.

### Hour 6 (Noon)

Prepare your lunch from the Pain-Control Menu or create a lunch plan of your own based on it. Remember that fast foods could be pain foods, so take the time to "cook for freedom from pain" with healthful ingredients. Take your DLPA and L-tryptophan.

### Hour 7 (1:00 P.M.)

Repeat your back, neck, and shoulder exercises plus your six-second movie of the mind. Follow with a biofeedback exercise. It's not only relaxing in itself, it reaffirms that the new therapy for chronic pain relief is working for you.

### Hours 8 to 10 (2:00 to 4:00 P.M.)

Get back into the world again. Meet with a friend at your home or his or hers. Don't talk about your pain, talk about your recovery from pain (among other things). Your friend's admiration for your determination to stay on your pain-control program will strengthen your resolve to do so. It's a good idea to take a short walk with your friend during this period. Excuse yourself at about Hour 9 (3:00 P.M.) to perform your exercises and movie of the mind.

### Hours 11 to 13 (5:00 to 7:00 P.M.)

If you have children returning from school, spend some time with them; after a while, show off your improvement in a natural unaffected way by starting to prepare dinner. They'll be happy to help you, and that will provide a lift to your spirits that also helps ease your pain. Around Hour 12 (6:00 P.M.), perform a total relaxation technique. You'll be relaxed and refreshed and feeling a minimum amount of pain when your spouse returns from work. Now there's another hand to help prepare and serve dinner and assist with the cleaning up afterward. Before dinner, repeat your exercises and six-second movie of the mind.

### Hour 13 (7:00 P.M.)

Dinner is a selection from the Pain-Control Menu or variations suggested by you and the rest of the family. The dinner can be the same for all. Dinnertime is the most important meal of the day for you psychologically. It is the time for family communications and the cementing of interrelations. It is the time for you to practice everything you've learned about changing you and your family's attitudes toward pain.

### Hours 14 to 17 (8:00 to 11:00 P.M.)

After dinner, repeat your exercises and movie of the mind. Settle down with your spouse for an evening of conversation, TV watching, reading, or games. If you feel up to it have some friends in occasionally. At around 9:30, repeat your exercises and movie of the mind. Just before bedtime, perform a total relaxation technique and take your DLPA and L-tryptophan.

### Hours 18 through 24 (11:00 P.M. to 7 A.M.)

There's no reason why you can't enjoy sex. It could help relieve your pain. You've had a full day, you're relaxed, your pain is way down, you're happy with the way things are going. You'll sleep soundly.

## YOUR PAIN-CONTROL
## PROGRAM TIMETABLE

As you learn each new pain-control technique from Chapters 5 through 12, enter it on a time slot on the following chart. Use the preceding Hour-by-Hour Chronic-Pain-Control Program as a model. Confer with the physician supervising this program to be sure you have made the correct placement. Should supplementary outpatient or clinical therapies be advised, enter them on Your Pain-Control Timetable as well.

*Check off the following techniques as you enter them.* The list looks long and formidable, but don't let it frighten you. You don't eat a steak in one gulp, you eat it bite by bite. Add one technique at a time, as soon as you're comfortable with it. Exceptions: Start at once to eat right (Chapter 9), change your family's attitude toward pain (Chapter 11), and take your DLPA and L-tryptophan (Chapter 8). You should start breaking your drug habit from the beginning, with the help of your supervising physician. Often, the patient won't get better until he or she starts coming off drugs. Remember, you don't *have* to use every technique—just the ones you and your physician decide are right for you.

| | | |
|---|---|---|
| Start now | ☐ | Your pain-control diet (page 107) |
| Start now | ☐ | Changing your family's attitude toward pain (page 127) |
| Start now | ☐ | DLPA and L-tryptophan (pages 95, 99) |
| Start now | ☐ | Your get-going exercises (page 41) |
| Start now | ☐ | Your keep-going exercises (page 43) |
| | ☐ | A basic exercise for lower back pain (page 51) |
| | ☐ | A basic exercise for musculoskeletal pains (page 51) |
| | ☐ | Exercises you can do away from home (page 51) |

Start at
least one
now
{
□ Deep breathing (page 57)
□ Conditioned relaxation (page 58)
□ Transcendental meditation (page 59)
□ Biofeedback (page 60)
□ Autogenics (page 68)
□ Self-hypnosis (page 68)
□ Movies of the mind (page 85)

Start now □ Breaking the narcotic analgesic/sedative drug habit (page 116)

## THE FUTURE YOU

After several months on this regimen, you may be fit for your job again (homemaking is a job, too), and for your regular life. Your pain may shrink to a small fraction of its former potency or vanish entirely.

Plan to *keep* pain away. Continue to exercise daily—do your morning bed exercises and your back, neck, and shoulder exercises at least once a day. Add walking or swimming, or another form of aerobic exercise, to your lifestyle. Stay on your pain-control diet. Include your twenty-minute total relaxation technique in your daily schedule.

Should pain return, resume your hour-by-hour chronic-pain-control program at once, and consult the physician who supervised it. But most of all, don't worry. You've beaten pain once. This time, it will be easier. And perhaps this time will be the last time.

# YOUR PAIN-CONTROL PROGRAM TIMETABLE

|  | Your Time | Your Daily Pain-Control Activity |
|---|---|---|
| Hour 1 | _____ | _____ |
| Hour 2 | _____ | _____ |
| Hour 3 | _____ | _____ |
| Hour 4 | _____ | _____ |
| Hour 5 | _____ | _____ |
| Hour 6 | _____ | _____ |
| Hour 7 | _____ | _____ |
| Hour 8 | _____ | _____ |
| Hour 9 | _____ | _____ |
| Hour 10 | _____ | _____ |
| Hour 11 | _____ | _____ |
| Hour 12 | _____ | _____ |
| Hour 13 | _____ | _____ |
| Hour 14 | _____ | _____ |
| Hour 15 | _____ | _____ |
| Hour 16 | _____ | _____ |
| Hour 17 | _____ | _____ |
| Hour 18 | _____ | _____ |
| Hour 19 | _____ | _____ |
| Hour 20 | _____ | _____ |
| Hour 21 | _____ | _____ |
| Hour 22 | _____ | _____ |
| Hour 23 | _____ | _____ |
| Hour 24 | _____ | _____ |

# 13

# How to Adapt
# Your Pain-Control Program
# to Your Type of Pain

Your pain-control program has been designed to treat any kind of chronic pain. For some kinds of pain, certain elements of the program are emphasized for maximum pain control. This chapter will tell you what those elements are for the treatment of headache pain, backache pain, arthritis pain, angina pain, musculoskeletal pain, and other types of pain. You will also become acquainted with some supplementary treatments that have proved to be helpful in some cases.

## HEADACHE PAIN

Headaches are not regarded as a disease per se but rather as symptoms of underlying disorders. Removal of the disorders should remove the headaches. Prevention of the disorders should prevent the headaches. But if headache care were that easy, 46 million Americans—about 80 percent of them women—wouldn't be suffering from headaches.

If you're one of that astounding multitude of headache sufferers and you haven't had a thorough medical evaluation, or if you've had a recent change for the worse, then by all means get a complete medical checkup. If, however, the diagnosis given to you is "migraine" or "cluster headache," "tension" or "muscle contraction headache," or "sinus headache," then you can expect relief.

You can get it through your pain-control program. For tension and migraine headaches, rely particularly on the total relaxation techniques, with heavy emphasis on biofeedback. For tension headaches, look especially to the good-posture exercise and the neck exercise (pages 48 and 47) as well as the total relaxation techniques.

Here are some additional specific ways you can get fast relief when your "head is splitting."

### Tension Headaches

These may be relieved with a specific movie of the mind. It is described by a young woman who no longer suffers from persistent tension headaches.

*My pain is a naked light bulb. It's in the middle of my head. It's big. It's 500 watts. The glare is strong, as strong as my pain. I see a knob, the kind that you turn to make a light less bright. I turn the knob. Slowly. Very slowly. I know this is going to take minutes. I can see the light beginning to dim. It's getting dimmer and dimmer. As it does, the glare shrinks in the bulb. The glare gets smaller and smaller. Dimmer and dimmer. Smaller and smaller, Dimmer and dimmer. The light shrinks to the size of a marble . . . a pea . . . a pinpoint. Then it goes out. As it goes out, so does my pain.*

The neck exercises in Chapter 4 are also particularly useful.

### Migraine Headaches

Be careful to avoid the pain-inducing foods listed on page 106. They are particularly dangerous to chronic-migraine sufferers. Lying down in a quiet dark room helps; a researcher for this book, who has suffered from migraine since age ten, aborts migraine attacks by doing just that the instant the typical migraine aura strikes. (The aura is a dazzling display of zigzagging lights before one eye or both.) The pain of migraine may also be diminished somewhat by scalp and/or neck massage, finger pressure on the painful area, and cold compresses. Autogenics, self-hypnotic suggestion of hand-warming, and biofeedback can all be extremely helpful.

### Other Types of Headaches

There are about fifty-five types of headaches. Of these, the most common, besides tension and migraine, are cluster and sinus headaches.

- *Cluster headaches,* which, as the name denotes, come in clusters, are a severe form of vascular headache. They respond as migraine does, to your pain-control program and to the added pain-control measures suggested in this section.
- *Sinus headaches* can also be helped by your pain-control program. These headaches can be relieved by eliminating the cause, which may be sinus infection, a condition due to allergies, or blockage of sinus drainage.

It is wise, while you're obtaining rapid relief from your headache, no matter what kind, to have your doctor investigate its origins. Getting to the source of your headaches, and treating the source, is the preferable way to end headache pain permanently. Stress is often a source, and alleviating stress could help prevent many types of headaches, certainly tension headaches. The total relaxation techniques and the exercises given in your pain-control program could, therefore, be a potent headache-prevention therapy.

## BACKACHE PAIN

You should perform the exercises given on pages 45–49 daily if you are a victim of backache—and you may very well be since, after the common cold, it is the most prevalent malady in America.

The physician supervising your pain-control program will help you determine just how much exercise is right for you.

Bed rest may hasten recovery of simple backache due to strain of muscles and ligaments, but it should be kept short—two days at most. Many pain-control specialists are now recommending to victims of backache as early a return to work or to active home-making as possible, even if they are feeling some pain. Recent studies demonstrate that simple backache will go away in a week or two with minimum, or even no, bed rest. Activity is not apt to result in further injury.

It is likely that curtailing or eliminating bed rest helps relieve the three D's—depression, dependence, and disability—associated with painful conditions of any kind. Moreover, extended bed rest may cause loss of muscular strength, be harmful to the circulatory system, and create an adverse psychological state resulting from loss of freedom.

On the other hand, if your backache is caused by ruptured disks or nerve damage, longer bed rest may be mandatory. Even in these cases, bed rest can be overdone, and eventually exercise is almost always necessary for recovery. Consult your doctor if you're in doubt about the best treatment for you.

## ARTHRITIS PAIN

The odds are 1 in 7 that you are an arthritis victim; 36 million Americans are. Your arthritis may have been diagnosed as rheumatoid arthritis or osteoarthritis, the two most common forms, or as bursitis, systemic lupus erymatosis, ankylosing spondylitis, or any of about one hundred different varieties. The pain of all can be diminished through your pain-control program. Emphasis should be placed on exercise, diet, and movies of the mind.

Exercises are best done after the acute phase of red, swollen, and hot joints has quieted down. The best exercises for arthritis involve the arms, the legs, the neck, and the upper body. You'll find suitable ones on pages 47–50. They help restore frozen joints to mobility and keep them flexible. Also, try to walk as much as possible.

If you're overweight—and many arthritis sufferers are—use the pain-control diet as a reducing diet. Follow the instructions in Chapter 10. Reducing to ideal weight has been associated with relief of arthritic pain. The diet is the type recommended in the Federal Dietary Guidelines to fight degenerative diseases, including arthritis. There is some evidence that only fish with high concentrations of EPA—ecosopentanoic acid—have antiinflammatory properties. For example; salmon, herring, mackeral, and tuna.

There is also some evidence that the nutrient DLPA, which is used in your pain-control program to fight depression and pain, can also be effective in reducing the inflammation of arthritis, particularly osteoarthritis. A somewhat higher dosage than that suggested for the pain-control program may be prescribed by your physician.

An excellent movie of the mind is to see your joints as you want to see them. The following is such a movie, created by a sixty-year-old woman who suffered from rheumatoid arthritis.

*My hands are healthy. They're beautiful, healthy hands. Nothing's wrong with them. Can I move them again? I try. One finger. It moves. Another. It moves. I try all the fingers of my hands, one after another. They all move. Can I use them again without pain? I pick up a skillet. No pain. I open a can. No pain. I knit. No pain. I take my violin out of its case. I hold it under my chin. I touch the bow to it. I play a wild gypsy dance. I play on and on and on, faster and faster and faster.*

For additional temporary relief, try warm or cold compresses and warm baths.

## ANGINA PAIN

This pain is associated with clogged arteries that starve the heart of blood. It is the pain of atherosclerosis and heart attack. If you're not already a victim of this frightening pain, chances are that you will be. Shockingly, one out of two Americans will experience the pain of angina sometime in their lives.

On your pain-control program, it's a manageable pain, particularly because of the exercise plan, diet, and total relaxation techniques.

The aerobic exercise plan is designed to increase blood flow to all parts of the body, especially the heart. It's wise, under the supervision of your physician, to supplement the exercises with walking (slowly at first, then briskly), then jogging, and, eventually, even running. Once you've reached the right stage of physical fitness, swimming is an excellent way to help prevent angina, as are dancing, tennis, and climbing stairs. But your exercise must be regular, within the limits of your physical capacity, and doctor-approved.

Your pain-control diet is, perhaps, the perfect diet for fighting the underlying causes of angina. Based on dietary recommendations of the American Heart Association and the American Dietetic Association, the diet eliminates or reduces to acceptable levels all the nutrients indicted by modern medical science as mainly responsible for the atherosclerotic conditions associated with angina. We strongly recommend that this diet be followed rigorously.

Total relaxation techniques lower stress. Performed daily, these techniques help you cope with the stress of pain and of everyday life. When you eliminate that stress you eliminate a trigger of angina attacks.

## MUSCULOSKELETAL PAIN

This stress-related pain of muscles, bone, and the physiological connections between them, is treated in your pain-control program with emphasis on exercise and total relaxation techniques.

This pain-control treatment helps break the "musculoskeletal pain cycle," which now traps some 40 million Americans. It is a cycle that begins with pain (sometimes stress-induced, sometimes injury-induced) that tenses the muscles, causing anxiety, which increases muscle tension, which increases pain, which further tenses the muscles, which raises the anxiety, which intensifies the pain . . . and round and round in a vicious cycle of pain. With your pain-control program, you break the cycle by relieving muscle tension mainly through exercise and total relaxation techniques.

Additional help for musculoskeletal pain—particularly of the lower back, neck and shoulders, hip and knee—may come from acupuncture and TENS (see page 155), when recommended by the physician supervising your program. Massage, which has a calming effect and is a pleasing antidote to stress, is also an option, especially for the pain of muscle spasms.

## OTHER PAINS

In mild or moderate cases of *cancer,* or in cases of neurogenic pains, especially face pains, the emphasis in your pain-control program is on total relaxation techniques and movies of the mind.

For the pain of *sciatica,* autogenics may be stressed.

*Stomach pain* may yield especially to total relaxation techniques, especially when the stomach is cleared of such irritants as aspirin, coffee, tea, cola drinks, and alcohol.

*Kidney and urinary pain* therapy may center on movies of the mind.

Biofeedback is a powerful technique for the treatment of *all pain.* Acupuncture may be an effective supplement to your pain-control program.

In addition, for each kind of pain there are traditional non-drug treatments, including compresses, massages, water therapy (baths, Jacuzzi), heat, ice, and pressure, which you should explore with your physician. There's every reason to add them to your program if there's a good-to-excellent chance they'll help speed your recovery.

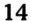

# 14

# New Hope Therapies
# for a Pain-Control Program

The assumption throughout this book has been that the program outlined here is part of a larger, ongoing program of medical care. To round out the picture, then, I think it is useful to discuss other therapies available to you at pain-control clinics and how you might choose among the clinics themselves. Some clinics are better than others; we can feel comfortable recommending some therapies now, but others we cannot.

## NEW HOPE THERAPIES
## THAT CAN SUPPLEMENT
## YOUR PAIN-CONTROL PROGRAM

### Acupuncture

James Reston was a highly respected and much-honored columnist of the *New York Times.* In 1971, after his appendix was removed at a hospital in Peking, China, he suffered from severe postoperative gas pains. The doctors at the hospital inserted stainless steel needles—hair-thin, with a rounded point to push aside tissue, not cut it—into Reston's . . . stomach? No, into his knees and at his right elbow.

"It was a rather complicated way to get rid of gas in the stomach," Reston said. "But there was a noticeable relaxation of the pressure and distension within an hour and no recurrence of the problem thereafter."

James Reston had been cured by a Chinese therapy more than two thousand years old—acupuncture. Inserted at body points indicated on traditional Chinese acupuncture charts—points almost never near, almost always far from, the site of the pain—the needles, carefully twirled for several seconds, have been claimed by Chinese doctors to be routine procedure for minor cures and miracles. Disbelieved, scorned, and rejected by American doctors, acupuncture was put to the test beginning one year after Reston's *Times* story had blitzed the nation by one of the great pioneers in the new pain-control therapy, Dr. David E. Bressler.

Bressler, a hard-nosed skeptic, had been influenced in his decision to conduct a scientific investigation of acupuncture by a demonstration he had witnessed in the clinic of Los Angeles acupuncturist, Master Ju Gim Shek. The patient, Dr. Bressler recounts, "was a man in his late sixties . . . with osteoarthritis in both hands. His knuckles were swollen to the size of walnuts, and he complained of such agonizing pain that it was difficult even to examine him."

Most of the needles were placed at points that were remote from the knuckles—in the patient's back, ears, and feet. The closest needles were pressed into his hands, but not his knuckles. After two minutes of needle manipulation by Ju, the patient, reports Bressler, "exclaimed, 'My God, the pain is gone. It's a miracle.'" He told Bressler that he hadn't felt the needles at all. "'I feel wonderful all over. This is the first time in fifteen years that I don't have pain.'"

"The guy must be a nut," Dr. Bressler later admitted thinking. "He's crazy. He still has pain; he just *thinks* he doesn't have pain." (Bressler's emphasis)

But after Bressler's shock wore off, he objectively compared Ju's therapy with the best American medicine could offer at that time— "'Get the largest jar of aspirin you can find and eat one every four hours'; or worse, 'Nothing can be done; you'll just have to learn to live with it'"—and concluded that a clinical study of acupuncture was in order.

The result of Dr. Bressler's eight-year study, undertaken at the UCLA Pain-Control Unit, where he is still the director, clearly established acupuncture as a potent therapeutic tool, but not a panacea, when integrated in a total pain-control program. He found the ancient Chinese remedy effective not only in osteoarthritic cases like the one he saw treated by Ju, but also in low back, neck and shoulder, hip and knee pains, trigeminal (tic) and other neuralgias, and tension and migraine headaches. Our experience at the Pain Alleviation Center parallels Dr. Bressler's.

No one knows how acupuncture works, but the popular theory is that the acupuncture points act as buttons to the pain-control center of the brain, and pressure on them opens a flow of endorphins. Some experiments have, indeed, demonstrated that brain endorphin levels rise after acupuncture.

Can you incorporate acupuncture into your pain-control program? Not if you try to do it yourself, even though finger pressure can produce the needle effect in some cases. Too little is known here about this still-strange therapy to be deemed useful or safe in the hands of a nonprofessional.

But if acupuncture is approved by your physician, you may benefit from the help of a trained and experienced acupuncturist to whom you're referred. Such professionals are on the staff of most pain-control centers, including ours. In California and New York, an applicant must provide proof of extensive training and pass a rigorous examination to obtain a license to practice acupuncture—a procedure other states are likely to follow.

It's wise to scrutinize the credentials of any acupuncturist whom you are thinking of engaging.

## Electrical Stimulation

Endorphin production, it now appears, may be stimulated by brief pulses of electricity applied to nerve endings through the skin, known in medical parlance as *transcutaneous electrical nerve stimulation* (TENS). Results like those recorded by Dr. C. Norman Shealy, director of the Pain and Rehabilitation Center, La Crosse, Wisconsin, in a pioneering study—significant pain relief in 132 out of 136 chronic-pain patients—have been roughly replicated in other clinics.

The electrical pulses are generated by a small machine, which can be worn on your belt. Wires from it lead to tiny electrodes, which are attached with adhesive tape to the skin at the sites of pain. The machine is adjustable to provide the right voltage and frequency of pulsation for individual requirements.

There are several advantages of TENS. It can be turned on at any time, day or night, to provide instant relief. It is nonaddictive, generally safe for short-term use when physicians' instructions are followed, and not expensive. It provides that important feeling of being in control which most chronic-pain patients have lost. There are no adverse side effects.

But there are several disadvantages, the most serious of which is that you may rapidly develop a tolerance to the pulses, and unless you're on a total pain-control program you're back at square one, disappointed and disheartened. Other disadvantages are minor: the possibility of skin burns if the machine is not adjusted properly, some difficulty in attaching the apparatus, and the embarrassment of appearing in public wearing a therapeutic machine.

TENS has been a successful component of our total pain-control program at the Pain Alleviation Center. It is particularly effective in the treatment of neck, shoulder, and back pains originating in the muscles attached to the skeletal structure. Should you include TENS in your pain-control program? If your physician recommends it, yes, but never without medical approval and supervision.

There are two other types of electrical stimulation, both involving surgery: *brain stimulation,* also known as stimulation-produced analgesia (SPA), and *dorsal column stimulation* (DCS).

In brain stimulation, a remote-control electronic device (like the one for your TV set) activates a receiver under the skin, which sends electrical impulses along wires connected to electrodes surgically implanted in the brain. The electrodes are placed in brain sites rich in endorphin-producing cells, which are intensely stimulated by the electrical shocks.

Patients who have used this technique, particularly for the gruesome pain of advanced cancer, report that their pain "seems to melt away." They also state that their brain is sharp and clear after the therapy, as contrasted with the muddled confusion they had experienced with strong analgesic drugs.

But brain stimulation is fraught with the intrinsic hazard of brain surgery. It is expensive. And what is heartbreakingly discouraging, some patients develop a tolerance of the electrical input, and after repeated treatments the pain returns as strongly as or stronger than before.

This last-resort treatment is not part of your pain-control program. You should agree to its use only after consultation with a pain-control specialist and a neurosurgeon trained and experienced in the technique.

In dorsal column stimulation, a small radio receiver is surgically implanted under the skin close to the spine, and two electrodes attached to it are connected to the back (the dorsal side) of the spinal column. The radio is activated to send electrical impulses into the dorsal column by a hand-held antenna attached to a small battery-operated radio transmitter hanging on the patient's belt. The patient waves the antenna, much like a magic wand, over the site of the under-skin radio receiver to relieve his or her pain.

Creators of dorsal column stimulation, Dr. C. Norman Shealy and Dr. Blaine S. Nashville, of the Pain and Rehabilitation Center, La Crosse, Wisconsin, claim success in treating a wide range of pains, including the pain of cancer. Whether the electrical impulses block the transmission of pain impulses through the nerves of the spinal cord, or whether they stimulate the production of endorphins, or whether some still unknown pain-control mechanism is involved, is not yet understood.

Unfortunately, tolerance to the effects of dorsal column stimulation can also develop. In addition, the electrodes sometimes move and have to be repositioned surgically. Infection is a risk, as with any surgical procedure. This is another last-resort therapy that should be undertaken only on the basis of sound medical advice. It is not a component of your pain-control program.

## The Placebo Effect

Can a sugar pill stop your pain? Can an injection of salt water? They did—even after major surgery—in a remarkable 35 percent of chronic-pain patients tested. Obtaining relief from a substance with no therapeutic properties is known as the placebo effect, and for the first time in medical history it is under in-depth investigation by expert medical teams.

The use of the placebo, which probably goes back to the beginnings of medicine, originated with the doctors' need to please the patients for whom they had no medicine that worked. (*Placebo* is Latin for "I shall please.") An intended harmless deception, it often turned out, much to the doctors' surprise, to be an effective therapeutic tool.

But the reasons behind the success baffled them. Suggestion? Distraction? Optimism? Hope? Too vague to satisfy hard-headed scientists. But now, thanks to a remarkable experiment conducted with the support of the National Institute of Neurological and Communicative Disorders and Strokes, medical investigators at the University of California at San Francisco, seem to have found the answer.

Adults scheduled for wisdom-tooth removal, a major dental surgical procedure with which severe postoperative pain is associated, were asked to volunteer to test the effectiveness of pain-control drugs. Some patients were given morphine, some a placebo.

About one third of the patients given the placebo showed no signs of pain.

They were then given naloxone, a drug that blocks the brain's use of its endorphins. All of the placebo-pain-free patients then felt pain.

The investigators made the obvious conclusion: The placebo stimulated the production of endorphins.

But how? There was nothing in the placebo to do it. The only viable explanation is that the placebo triggered the patients' access to the unconscious part of the brain that may control endorphin flow. Simply stated: If you feel deeply that something is going to work for you, your unconscious brain will make it work for you.

Why didn't the placebo effect work for two thirds of the subjects? The investigators suspect that stress makes the difference. The unaffected were the cool, calm, and collected types. The affected were stressed. Why stress makes communication with the unconscious mind easier is puzzling.

What does the placebo effect mean to you on your pain-control program? A great deal. It's the basic principle behind the technique developed at the Pain Alleviation Center for weaning you from analgesic drugs, which was explained in Chapter 11 (page 127).

## Behavior Modification

Chronic pain is not only a life-altering phenomenon, it's a life*style*-altering one. A chronic-pain sufferer becomes a different person: A different person is one who behaves differently; a person who behaves differently is one with a new lifestyle.

What is the lifestyle of the pained and miserable?

You may be living parts of the worst possible scenario, or all of it, right now. If you are, it's bad for you. It works against your improvement. It encourages you—as incredible as it sounds—to cling to your pain. We at the Pain Alleviation Center, see patients to whom pain becomes a welcome friend. Tragically, they do not realize what has happened to them until we point it out. Only then are they open to treatment by behavior modification to change their lifestyle. Follow this sad scenario of the lifestyle of a chronic-pain sufferer, Harry Townsend, and if it resembles yours in any way, it's time for you to practice behavior modification.

Before chronic pain struck, Harry was a nobody. He worked as a bill collector, a low-echelon job that brought him no respect. He was forty and looked older, paunchy, and balding. He was the butt of family jokes, even from his children. Because he was unable to bully delinquent debtors in the course of his work, he was a pushover for any assertive person. He saw himself as a wimp to whom nobody paid any attention.

But pain made him the center of attention. Everybody said, "Poor Harry, what can I do for you?" It gave him a wonderful sense of power. "Oh, my sciatica is killing me. Please do . . ." Whatever it was, his wife, children, friends, and relatives would hop to it. He found that the more he complained, the more attention he got, so he complained more. Harry wasn't faking; the pain was real, and it was getting worse. But he was using it to manipulate people, not deliberately, not maliciously, perhaps unconsciously, but gratifyingly.

Harry's pain was so bad that he had to give up his job, which he had hated anyway. He had hated having to struggle to meet his bills on a paycheck depleted by deductions. But now, with disability insurance and company and government benefits, he was earning more than he had been when he was working, and without deductions. Harry was a man of leisure, without a financial worry in the world. Sometimes he wondered what would happen if his pain ever stopped. Back to work? Back to struggling with the bills? His pain didn't stop.

When his wife said, "Harry, I want you to talk to the children because they're getting out of hand," Harry would say, "Not now, honey. I'm in too much pain." What a great way Harry had discovered to duck responsibility. He could flee from disagreeable confrontations and avoid making unpleasant decisions—any decisions, except those that had to do with his own desires. Harry had considered himself a failure in everything he had done all his adult life, but now he couldn't fail. He would never again be in a win-lose situation. Thanks to his pain, he was out of the daily battle.

There was a downside to Harry's new lifestyle. To make people believe he was in pain, he had to show pain. Let people get the idea that the pain was only in his head, or that he was exaggerating or putting them on, and his new lifestyle would be smashed. So anxiety invaded Harry's life; to rid himself of it and quell his fears of losing everything he had gained, he put on a better show of pain. He became homebound, spent more time in bed, grew more dependent on his family. He popped more pills, had his family take him to his doctor more often, and even underwent surgery. But there was no end to the pain.

Harry did not *plan* this scenario—it's most unlikely that any chronic-pain sufferer does—but once the first change in lifestyle occurs, the rest seems to be inevitable.

Harry was rehabilitated by behavior modification. A psychological technique aimed at eliminating dependence on pain as a way of life, it opens the way to a successful treatment of pain. It is designed to break unwholesome behavior patterns of chronic-pain sufferers by encouraging the very opposite of those behaviors: independence instead of dependence, responsibility instead of irresponsibility, activity instead of lethargy, and the desire to free oneself from pain and not be bound to it.

In practice, reversing the chronic-pain lifestyle can be accomplished only by putting yourself in the hands of expert psychologists trained and experienced in pain care. Rewarding the patient for positive changes in lifestyle, and withholding rewards for not making these changes, is the core of the behavior modification (technical name: operant conditioning) technique. The rewards are praise and attention.

If your supervising physician and a psychotherapist, having made a complete assessment of your style of life, should decide that you are a candidate for behavior modification, you could be helped by formal therapy.

If you do not undertake that therapy, you can fight the lure of the chronic-pain lifestyle by taking a yes attitude toward life.

Do I want to lick my pain? *Yes!*
Do I want to be independent? *Yes!*
Do I want to accept responsibility? *Yes!*
Do I want to be active? *Yes!*
Do I want to break reliance on drugs? *Yes!*
Do I want to go back to real life? *Yes!*
Do I want to feel proud of myself? *Yes!*
Do I want to lick my pain? *Yes!*

You can include your yesses to life without pain in your pain-control program. Just recite them at the start of each day and several times during your day. If you succeed in taking a *yes* attitude toward life, you will receive the same rewards as you would get on a behavior modification program: praise and attention. But you won't get them from psychotherapists; you'll get them from the people whom you love most and who love you most, your spouse and your children—and that's the best kind of praise and attention. Don't risk having them withhold those rewards.

## Counseling

The aim of this psychological technique for pain control is, like that of behavior modification, to alter your attitudes and feelings toward pain and your pain-induced behavior patterns. An important element of counseling is that it includes your family as well, because psychotherapists have established that the way those close to you view the you-in-pain could help bring about your recovery or prolong your misery.

Counseling may probe for hidden memories that accentuate your pain (Is it punishment for some childhood misdemeanor?), or motives (Whom else do you want to punish?). Counseling may involve an examination of your upbringing (Were those members of your family who were in pain given preferential treatment?), of your relations with others, past and present (Is your spouse really helping you?), and of your lifestyle (Does your job, literally, give you a pain?). Counseling may review your sex life (Is the fear of sex holding back your cure?). Counseling may involve your family (Are they standing firmly behind your rehabilitation efforts?) and your spiritual adviser (Do you lack faith that you can be helped?).

Counseling may be administered on a one-to-one basis or in a group. It is a standard element of the program at the Pain Alleviation Center and at most other advanced pain-control clinics. Your physician can refer you to a pain-control counselor should your condition necessitate it.

## Trigger-point Injections

Trigger points are distinct areas of muscle and other soft-tissue tenderness which can "trigger" pain at a distant site when they are pressed. Trigger point injections are done at the site of the "trigger," and relieve the pain elsewhere. The injections usually contain lidocaine or another, long-acting local anesthetic. They may also contain anti-inflammatory drugs such as cortisone. Trigger-point injections can be useful as part of an overall pain-control program, especially if followed by physical therapy.

# NEW HOPE THERAPIES
# THAT NEED FURTHER INVESTIGATION

## Shiatsu

This is a technique for applying deep pressure, usually by the thumb, to acupuncture points. It's a do-it-yourself, needleless form of acupuncture. Shiatsu (Japanese for "finger pressure") and two similar techniques, *do-In* and *tsubo,* are popular in Japan for creating a state of deep relaxation and managing chronic and other difficult-to-control medical problems. All these techniques, known collectively in this country as *acupressure,* have not yet been adequately tested by Western medicine.

## Somatic Therapy

*Somatic* means "pertaining to the body," and somatic therapists hold that just as the mind can direct the body, so the body can direct the mind. At the heart of the somatic theory is that stress and emotional problems, and disease and pain, so affect our musculature that our bodies move in unnatural fixed patterns. These convey a message to the brain that perpetuates and intensifies the original traumas, including pain. A restoration of natural body motions, through gentle physical manipulation, is claimed to send an opposite message to the brain, one which brings on a return of relaxation and emotional security, health, and the end of chronic pain.

But our bodies will sink back into distorted motions if we permit negative thoughts to hold sway over our minds, exponents of somatic therapy assert. "When we think the same thoughts of revenge over and over again," observes Thomas Hanna, director of the Novato Institute for Somatic Research and Training, San Francisco, "we are [harmfully] activating the muscles . . . of our bodies over and over again. When we repeat the same thought of disappointment over and over, we are repeatedly stamping its motor power into the tissues of our body until they sag in forlornness. When we repeatedly think with thoughts or memories of hurt, despair, anger or fear, we are physically injuring ourselves; we are engaged in self-destruction." One result, says Hanna, is pain, "the body's 'cry' to get back to normal."

In practice, somatic therapy is claimed to work through the use of a system of light "touches" (repositioning trauma-frozen muscles into natural positions for spontaneous action) devised by Moishe Feldenkrais, founder of the most popular form of somatic therapy, functional integration. But contrasted with the gentle Feldenkrais method is the deep-pressure tissue-manipulation massage of "Rolfing," a somatic therapy invented by Ida P. Rolf. Extremely painful during its application, this technique, which has the same aim as that of Feldenkrais, is said to produce deep relaxation and relief of pain immediately following the exercise. Neither Feldenkrais or Rolf is a doctor.

The reported success of somatic therapy (one of the researchers for this book witnessed the remarkable rehabilitation of a chronic-pain victim through Rolfing) has not been confirmed by extensive medical tests. Until it is, it would not be prudent to include it in your pain-control program. But a related therapy, "movement therapy," "therapeutic touch" massage, and other hand motions that seem to restore muscle function and stimulate endorphin flow (perhaps by pressure on acupuncture points), may be helpful; they could be included in your program on the advice of your physician. Physical therapy is also an option. And exercise crafted to meet your at-home and away-from-home needs to relax tensed-up muscles *is* a part of your program.

Chiropractic therapy is based on a concept quite different from Feldenkrais's or Rolf's, but it could be considered a form of somatic therapy. On the theory that minute dislocations of the vertebrae (the bony units of the spine) exert sufficient pressure on the nerves to cause pain, the chiropractor rectifies the dislocations by hand pressure. Before becoming a chiropractic patient, talk it over with your physician. You will probably be told that the

American Medical Association characterizes chiropractic doctors as "an unscientific cult"; but if your condition warrants it, you may be referred to such a practitioner. When chiropractic manipulation does work, it is probably because muscles are placed under a sudden stretch which can break muscle spasms and allow them to relax.

### Hormone Pain Blockers

The discovery in 1986 by Dr. Solomon Snyder of Johns Hopkins University that a body biochemical, bradykinin (one of a group of amino acids that act on blood vessels, smooth muscles, and nociceptive nerve endings), is responsible for painful sensations whenever the skin or vital organs are cut or damaged has led Dr. John Stewart of the University of Colorado to develop a synthetic chemical that blocks the action of bradykinin, thus eliminating pain. However, it has not yet been clinically tested or approved by the FDA. As understanding of the biochemistry of pain develops, it is likely that similar discoveries could open new pathways toward the management, and eventual termination, of chronic pain.

## WHAT TO LOOK FOR
## IN A PAIN-CONTROL CENTER

"People with chronic pain," observes that division of the National Institutes of Health concerned with pain, the National Institute of Neurological and Communicative Disorders and Stroke (NINCDS), "have usually seen a family doctor and several other specialists as well. Eventually, they are referred to neurologists, orthopedists or neurosurgeons.

"The patient-doctor relationship is extremely important in dealing with chronic pain. Both patients and family members should seek out knowledgeable specialists . . . who understand full well how pain has come to dominate the patient's life and the lives of everyone else in the family.

"Many specialists today refer to chronic pain patients to pain clinics for treatment. Pain clinic patients . . . are men and women of all ages, education and social backgrounds, suffering a wide variety of painful conditions. . . . Patients with low back pain are frequent, and so are people with complications of diabetes, stroke, brain trauma, headache, arthritis, or any of the rarer pain conditions. . . . The majority of patients . . . usually report substantial improvement."

What should you look for in a pain-control clinic? Before you commit yourself to a course of treatment, find out from a ranking staff member the answers to the following questions.

|  | YES | NO |
|---|---|---|
| Is the center staffed with specialists in physical medicine and rehabilitation, physical therapy, exercise physiology, psychiatry, and psychology? | ☐ | ☐ |
| Do the specialists perform as a team to provide pain relief built on an integrated multifaceted approach? | ☐ | ☐ |
| Is the center well equipped, including biofeedback and physical therapy equipment, especially exercise machines? | ☐ | ☐ |
| Will I receive a comprehensive evaluation of my condition prior to treatment, including a physical examination, a psychological assessment, and a review of my medical records? | ☐ | ☐ |
| Are the results of my comprehensive evaluation review by the treatment team used to determine whether I'm a candidate for the pain-control center? | ☐ | ☐ |
| Will my degree of motivation be a factor in my acceptance as a patient? If my degree of motivation is low, will I be rejected? | ☐ | ☐ |

Will the treatment team work out a program for my particular needs? ☐ ☐

Will a member of the treatment team explain and discuss my program with me and my family? ☐ ☐

Will the treatment team meet regularly to discuss my progress and make changes in my program if necessary? ☐ ☐

Will I receive a face-to-face report from a member of the treatment team about my progress and any changes in my program? ☐ ☐

Will my treatment be coordinated with the doctor who referred me to the center? ☐ ☐

Will I be helped to change my and my family's attitudes to my pain? ☐ ☐

|  | YES | NO |
|---|---|---|
| Are all of the following therapies available? | | |
| Trigger-point injections | ☐ | ☐ |
| Nerve blocks | ☐ | ☐ |
| Transcutaneous electrical nerve stimulation (TENS) | ☐ | ☐ |
| Acupuncture | ☐ | ☐ |
| Biofeedback training | ☐ | ☐ |
| Total relaxation training | ☐ | ☐ |
| Self-hypnosis training | ☐ | ☐ |
| Guided imagery training | ☐ | ☐ |
| Physical therapy | ☐ | ☐ |
| Movement therapy | ☐ | ☐ |
| Individualized activity and exercise programs | ☐ | ☐ |
| Assertiveness training | ☐ | ☐ |
| Behavior modification/life enhancement group therapy | ☐ | ☐ |

| | | |
|---|---|---|
| Medication management aimed at eliminating habit-forming painkilling and sedative drugs | ☐ | ☐ |
| Nutrition and diet guidance | ☐ | ☐ |

If the answer to every question is yes, as it should be, the chances are high that you will receive these benefits from a pain-control center.

- You will learn new and effective techniques for reducing the frequency and intensity of your pain.
- You will learn that pain is not just a medical problem, but an interrelated emotional, social, and familial problem, and how to solve it.
- You will learn how to improve your overall health and fitness and attain your ideal weight.
- You will learn how to acquire positive attitudes toward your pain and how to switch your family's attitudes from negative to positive.
- You will learn how to raise your self-esteem.
- You will learn *about* pain, so you know what's happening to you and what to do about it.
- You will learn how to treat your pain without habit-forming narcotic analgesic and sedative drugs.

The aim of the pain-control center, NINCDS sums up, "is to reduce pain medication and so improve the patient's pain problem that when he or she leaves [the center] it is with the prospect of resuming normal activities with a minimal requirement for analgesics, and with a positive self-image."

# 15

# The Questions Most Frequently Asked About Chronic Pain

One of the aims of this book is to tell you everything you need to know about pain. I have tried to dispel the myths and misconceptions that have grown up around what pain is, and what you can do about it, and replace them with sound, practical data and techniques. You have a right to know the truth about pain as advanced pain-control specialists view it. There's no other way for you, in consultation with the physician supervising your pain-control program, to make reasonable decisions about your pain care.

In this chapter, I will round out your knowledge concerning your pain-control program and supplemental therapies—your *total* pain-control program—by answering the questions most frequently asked by our patients—questions that could very well be yours.

*I've had a normal physical exam, including X rays and other tests, but my doctor can find nothing wrong. Is my pain "in my head"?*

No, your pain is real. You're not hallucinating. You're not a mental case. Sometimes a physical cause can be identified with a new test called a thermogram. Sometimes the pain is caused by a malfunctioning of the "gate" in the spinal cord, which remains open, permitting pain messages to continue up the nerves of the spinal cord to the brain, when under normal circumstances it should be closed. Sometimes the cause of pain is a lack of endorphins, the brain's own painkillers. But whatever the cause, pain of "unknown origin" can be treated through a total pain-control program.

*I've heard that most doctors prescribe narcotic analgesics and sedatives for chronic pain. If that's standard practice, what's wrong with it?*

Narcotic analgesics (such as Darvon or compounds containing codeine, Talwin, Demerol, Percodan, and morphine), and sedatives (called sedative-hypnotics, they include Valium, Librium, Fiorinal, Dalmane, and barbiturates) *are* among the most widely prescribed therapeutic drugs in the world today. There's nothing wrong with prescribing them to alleviate acute pain and muscle spasm.

But these drugs are known to be *contraindicated* for chronic pain. They are not to be used because they can led to depression, chronic invalidism, addiction, adverse personality changes, and a worsening of the pain condition.

*I've heard on TV and elsewhere how hard it is to break any drug habit. I'm hooked on Percodan. Am I hooked on it for the rest of my life?*

Not if you don't want to be. We have developed a pain capsule regimen that, when used in a total pain-control program, lets you break the habit gradually with no withdrawal symptoms. You're not even aware when and by how much your drug dosage is being decreased. But when your Percodan (or any other narcotic analgesic drug) dosage *is* decreased, your pain is also decreased.

*I have a bad back, and I've been told by a few doctors that I have to live with the pain, that nothing can be done. Is that true?*

No, it's not. "Once a bad back, always a bad back" is a myth. You can relieve your pain through a total pain-control program. You don't have to live with any chronic pain, except, perhaps, that of advanced cancer—and even in that case some of the new pain-control therapies, such as guided imagery, may be helpful.

*I suffer from tension headaches, which I can't get rid of. Am I neurotic?*

No, you're not. Exposed to the high degree of stress that is the price of modern civilization, everybody is under tension, and a majority of us suffer from tension headaches. But they can be relieved through total pain-control programs, especially with total relaxation techniques.

*I suffer from migraine. I was told by my doctor that I should see a psychiatrist. Should I?*

Physical causes of migraine have been well documented, and the new techniques of a total pain-control program, such as biofeedback, treat it effectively. Psychiatry is not necessarily the answer.

*I suffer from chronic shoulder pain, and I want to get well. My family says I don't want to get well. That creates a great deal of tension. What can I do about it?*

First, examine yourself honestly. Maybe you like to cling to the special treatment you're getting, such as the money from the government and your insurance that comes in even though you're not working; and maybe you enjoy a life without working. Strangely, many chronic-pain sufferers find that their pain grants them a number of advantages, and they don't want to give them up. A total pain-control program gives you the opportunity of knowing yourself better and coming to a better relationship with your family.

*I have a "slipped disk." Surgery has been recommended. Should I agree to it?*

American surgeons are among the best in the world, and today's surgical techniques are unparalleled in medical history. But there is no surgery without risk, and one risk in surgery that aims to alleviate pain is that the pain will eventually return. The proper indications for surgery include a "progressive neurologic deficit," which means the impairment of your back is getting worse. When pain is the only symptom, surgery is often ineffective, and many conservative surgeons recommend non-surgical treatment. A safe, less expensive, noninvasive way to treat disk pain is through a total pain-control program.

*I tried self-hypnosis and it works. My doctor says that proves my pain is imaginary. Is she right?*

No. Just the reverse. In self-hypnosis you stimulate the brain's endorphins to go to work. They can go to work only on *real* pain.

*Should psychological chronic pain and physical chronic pain be treated differently?*

All pain is experienced in the mind and is therefore psychological. All chronic pain is also physical, in that there is usually some neurochemical disturbance, such as a probable decrease in endorphins, in addition to other bodily changes in hormones, soft tissue, and blood vessels. If these changes don't show up on our tests, which are often not sensitive enough to spot them, then the pain is sometimes labeled "psychological" or "not real."

The terms "psychological" and "physical" should be used to refer to the primary trigger for the pain: either depression and stress or some form of bodily injury or disease. However, both types of pain are experienced in the same way and probably involve the same neurochemical changes. The treatment described in this book therefore addresses all types of pain.

*Is it true that chronic pain is always a symptom that something in my body has been damaged?*

Sometimes, yes, as in the case of the so-called incurable diseases, like most cancers and forms of arthritis. But not always. Chronic pain can be brought on by depression and stress, which do not ordinarily qualify as "something wrong in the body."

Other forms of chronic-pain syndromes, such as myofascial pain condition, can cause pain and suffering without obvious underlying permanent damage. The flow of the endorphins, which has been diminished under those conditions, is restored to normal through a total pain-control program, and pain is consequently decreased.

*My doctor says he can't find a cause for my pain, but he's treating me anyhow. How can he, if he doesn't know the cause?*

He doesn't have to. If the treatment stimulates the production of endorphins, your pain can be alleviated, no matter what its cause. The stimulation of endorphin production is the key to the success of the total pain-control therapies.

*Is rest the best way to treat pain?*

Rest is *a* way if it's not abused. Prolonged bed rest can weaken muscles and encourage invalidism. It's better to get up and about, exercise, get involved in life. A total pain-control program stimulates endorphin production, in part, by encouraging activity.

*If the endorphins are such powerful pain killers, why can't I just take an endorphin pill or an injection?*

Endorphins in a pill would be destroyed by digestive juices. Endorphins have been synthesized in the laboratory only in experimental quantities and are not FDA-approved. Should they be approved, they would be extremely expensive, and they could be administered only through injection into the brain or spine, a potentially hazardous medical operation which would have to be repeated frequently.

*As a woman, am I more susceptible to pain than a man and therefore less likely to succeed on a total pain-control program?*

No, you're not more susceptible, nor are you less likely to succeed on such a program.

*I know somebody who went on a total pain-control program, and it didn't do her any good. Why?*

Not every patient succeeds, but most at the Pain Alleviation Center do. We are conducting an ongoing study to determine the causes of failure, with the objective of eliminating them. One thing is certain—those who succeed are highly motivated, sincerely want to get well, and stick rigorously to the day-in, day-out regimen.

*Can any doctor help me get rid of my chronic pain?*

Medicine is now highly specialized. A doctor trained and experienced in total pain-control therapy is best qualified to help you. To locate such a doctor, see page 165. However, most doctors can help you to relieve *acute* pain.

# Recommended Reading

This is a selection of some key publications in the field of chronic pain. Those preceded by an asterisk are meant for the lay reader as well as the professional. The others are scientific papers.

*Analgesia: How the Body Inhibits Pain Perception* by J. L. Mark. *Science* 195:471–73.

*Analgesia in Mice and Humans by D-phenylalanine* by R. Balagot, E. Ehrenpreis, K. Kubota, and J. Greenberg. *Advances in Pain Research and Therapy* 5:289–93.

\* *An Introduction to Electroanesthesia* by A. Limoge. Baltimore: University Park Press, 1975.

*Antagonism of Stimulation-produced Analgesia by Naloxone, a Narcotic Antagonist* by H. Akil, D. J. Mayer, and J. D. Liebeskind. *Science* 191:961–2.

\* *Autogenic Therapy,* W. Luthe, ed. New York: Grune & Stratton, 1969.

\* *Biofeedback* by M. T. Orne et al. Washington, D.C.: American Psychiatric Association, 1980–1.

*Biofeedback Therapy for Migraine* by J. L. Medina and M. A. Franklin. *Headache* 16:115–18.

*Chronic Low Back Pain,* M. Stauton-Hicks and R. A. Boas, eds. New York: Raven Press, 1982.

* *Chronic Pain: America's Hidden Epidemic* by S. E. Brena. New York: Atheneum/SMI, 1978.

* *Chronic Pain* by the U.S. Department of Health and Human Services, Public Health Service, National Institutes of Health. Bethesda, Maryland: NIH Publication No. 82-2406, April, 1982.

* *Clinical Hypnotherapy* by D. B. Cheek and L. M. LeCron. New York: Grune and Stratton, 1968.

* *Coping with Chronic Pain* by N. Hendler and J. A. Fenton. New York: Clarkson N. Potter, 1979.

*Diagnosis and Non-Surgical Management of Chronic Pain* by N. Hendler. New York: Raven Press, 1981.

* *Diet for a Small Planet* by F. Lappe. New York: Ballantine Books, 1971.

* *Directing the Movies of Your Mind* by A. Bry. New York: Harper and Row, 1978.

*DL-phenylalanine in Depressed Patients* by H. Beckman, M. A. Strauss, and E. Ludolph. *Journal of Neurological Transactions* 41:123–34.

* *DLPA to End Chronic Pain and Depression* by A. Fox and B. Fox. New York: Pocket Books, 1985.

*Effects of L- and D-Amino Acids on Analgesia* by E. C. Alleva, C. Castellano, and A. Olivera. *Brain Research* 198:249–52.

* *Endorphins, Brain Peptides that Act like Opiates* by R. Guillemin. *New England Journal of Medicine* 296:226–28.

*Endorphins in Chronic Pain* by B. G. L. Almay, F. Johannson, and L. V. Knorrin et al. *Pain* 5:153–162.

* *Endorphins, Profound Behavioral Effects* by F. E. Bloom. *Science* 194:630–34.

* *Families and Family Therapy* by S. Minuchin. Cambridge, Massachusetts: Harvard University Press, 1974.

* *Free Yourself from Pain* by D. E. Bresler. New York: Simon & Schuster/Fireside, 1979.

* *Healing by Electromagnetism—Fact or Fiction?* by R. Bentall. *New Scientist,* April 22, 1976, 166–67.

*Migraine Treated by Relaxation Therapy* by K. M. Hay and J. Madden. *Journal of the Royal College of General Practitioners* 21:664.

*Management of Myofascial Pain Syndrome in General Practice* by J. J. Bonica. *Journal of the American Medical Association* 164:732.

* *Mental Imagery* by A. Richardson. New York: Springer, 1969.

* *Musculoskeletal Pain* by D. A. Zohn and J. McMannell. Boston: Little, Brown, 1976.

*On the Language of Pain* by R. Melzack and W. S. Torgeson. *Anesthesiology* 34:50.

* *Pain Mechanisms; a New Theory* by R. Melzack and P. D. Wall. *Science* 150:971–79.

*Peptides in the Brain: The New Endocrinology of the Neuron* by R. Guilleman. *Science* 202:390–402.

* *Power Over Your Pain Without Drugs* by N. H. Olshan. New York: Beaufort Books, 1983.

* *Progressive Relaxation* by E. Jacobson. Chicago: University of Chicago Press, 1983.

* *Relieve Tension the Autogenic Way* by H. Lindeman. New York: Wyden, 1973.

*The Analgesic Activity of Human Beta-endorphin in Man* by Y. Hosobuchi and C. H. Yi. *Communications in Psychopharmacology* 2:33–37.

* *The Body of Life* by T. Hanna. New York: Knopf, 1980.

* *The Brain's Own Opiate* by R. Lewin. *New Scientist,* January, 1976.

*The Chronic Pain Patient* by P. C. Gildenberg and R. A. DeVaul. Basel, Switzerland: S. Karger, AG, 1973.

*The Chronic Pain Syndrome* by R. C. Black. *Surgical Clinic of North America* 55:(4) 999–1011.

* *The Conscious Brain* by S. Rose. London: Weidenfeld and Nicolson, 1973.

* *The Dieter's Gourmet Cookbook: Delicious Low-Fat, Low-Cholesterol Cooking and Baking Recipes Using No Sugar or Salt* by F. Prince. New York: Simon & Schuster/Fireside, 1979.

* *The Fabric of Mind* by Richard Bergland. Harmondsworth, England: Penguin, 1985.

*The Mechanism of Placebo Analgesia* by J. D. Levine, N. C. Gordon, and H. C. Field. *The Lancet* 282:654–57.

* *The Physiology of Meditation* by R. K. Wallace and H. Benson. *Scientific American,* February 1972, 84–90.

* *The Puzzle of Pain* by R. Melzack. New York: Basic Books, 1973.

* *The Relaxation Response* by H. Benson. New York: Morrow, 1975.

*The Transmission of Impulses from Nerve to Muscle* by B. Katz. *Proceedings of the Royal Society of London,* 155:455–77.

* *Therapeutic Exercise,* J. K. Basmajian, ed. Baltimore: Williams and Wilkins, 1978.

*Treatment of Pain by (percutaneous) Stimulation?* by W. H. Sweet and J. G. Wepsic. *Transactions of the American Neurological Association* 93:103–07.

# Index